1 MONTH OF FREE READING

at

www.ForgottenBooks.com

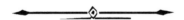

By purchasing this book you are eligible for one month membership to ForgottenBooks.com, giving you unlimited access to our entire collection of over 700,000 titles via our web site and mobile apps.

To claim your free month visit:

www.forgottenbooks.com/free163164

* Offer is valid for 45 days from date of purchase. Terms and conditions apply.

ISBN 978-0-267-16351-9
PIBN 10163164

This book is a reproduction of an important historical work. Forgotten Books uses state-of-the-art technology to digitally reconstruct the work, preserving the original format whilst repairing imperfections present in the aged copy. In rare cases, an imperfection in the original, such as a blemish or missing page, may be replicated in our edition. We do, however, repair the vast majority of imperfections successfully; any imperfections that remain are intentionally left to preserve the state of such historical works.

Forgotten Books is a registered trademark of FB &c Ltd.
Copyright © 2017 FB &c Ltd.
FB &c Ltd, Dalton House, 60 Windsor Avenue, London, SW19 2RR.
Company number 08720141. Registered in England and Wales.

For support please visit www.forgottenbooks.com

EPILEPSY

AND

OTHER CONVULSIVE AFFECTIONS;

THEIR

PATHOLOGY AND TREATMENT.

1822 - 1889

1858 London J. Church

220 2ed rev.

EPILEPSY

AND

OTHER CONVULSIVE AFFECTIONS,

THEIR

PATHOLOGY AND TREATMENT;

BY

CHARLES BLAND RADCLIFFE, M.D.,

PHYSICIAN TO THE WESTMINSTER HOSPITAL, ETC.

SECOND EDITION, REVISED AND ENLARGED.

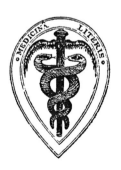

LONDON:

JOHN CHURCHILL, NEW BURLINGTON STREET.

MDCCCLVIII.

PREFACE.

In the former edition of this work I introduced the remarks I had to make upon epilepsy and other convulsive disorders by certain considerations respecting the physiology of muscular motion. I did this because I believed that there could be no satisfactory interpretation of those disorders in which muscular contraction is in excess until a radical error in the theory of muscular motion had been corrected. I knew of no better course then; I know of no better course now—for a sound physiology must ever go before a sound pathology. At the same time, it is at the option of any-one, who may so choose, to read the practical portion of this work first, and then to turn back and see how far the conclusions to which he is conducted by arguments of a purely pathological character—

arguments which are complete in themselves—are borne out by the physiology of muscular motion.

In treating of epilepsy and other convulsive affections, I trust that the thought and experience of the last four years will have enabled me to supply some of the deficiencies and to correct some of the errors which existed in the first edition. I do not propose, however, to enter into every part of the subject. On the contrary, I pass by several topics of considerable interest in themselves, but only of secondary importance in the argument, because I do not wish to divert attention from the object I have in view, which is to point out the necessity for a fundamental change in the pathology and treatment of the disorders under consideration—a change which is in accordance with that which would seem to be demanded in the physiology of muscular motion.

C. B. R.

4, HENRIETTA STREET,
   CAVENDISH SQUARE, W.

TABLE OF CONTENTS.

PRELIMINARY CONSIDERATIONS

RESPECTING THE

PHYSIOLOGY OF MUSCULAR MOTION.

	PAGE
Introductory remarks	1

I. *The First Proposition:—That muscular contraction is not produced by the stimulation of any property of contractility belonging to muscle* . . **9**

    1. That muscular contraction is not produced by the stimulation of electricity **9**
    2. That muscular contraction is not produced by the stimulation of "nervous influence" **39**
    3. That muscular contraction is not produced by the stimulation of the blood **65**
    4. That muscular contraction is not produced by the stimulation of any mechanical agent **79**
    5. That muscular contraction is not produced by the stimulation of light **88**
    6. That muscular contraction is not produced by the stimulation of heat or cold **89**
    7. That muscular contraction is not produced by the stimulation of any chemical or analogous agency . . **91**

	PAGE
II. *The Second Proposition:—That muscular elongation is produced by the simple physical action of certain agents, electricity and others, and that muscular contraction is the simple physical consequence of the cessation of this action*	100
III. *The Third Proposition:—That the special muscular movements which are concerned in carrying on the circulation—the rhythm of the heart and those movements of the vessels which are independent of the heart—are susceptible of a physical explanation when they are interpreted upon the previous view of muscular action*	114

EPILEPSY

AND

OTHER CONVULSIVE AFFECTIONS;

THEIR

PATHOLOGY AND TREATMENT.

Preliminary remarks . . 133

CHAPTER I.

OF SIMPLE EPILEPSY . 136

The general history of the epileptic .	136
The epileptic paroxysm .	142
The pathology .	156
The treatment	176

CHAPTER II.

OF TREMOR

PAGE 215

The history of tremor	215
Ordinary trembling	215
Paralysis agitans	216
Delirium tremens	216
The rigors and subsultus of fevers	217
The tremblings of slow mercurial poisoning	218
The pathology	218
The treatment	222

CHAPTER III.

OF SIMPLE CONVULSION

224

The general history of simple convulsion	224
Hysteric convulsion	224
Chorea	227
The paroxysm—	
Hysteric convulsion	231
Chorea	235
The dance of St. John	240
The dance of St. Vitus	241
Tarantism	243
The *Tigretier*	244
Cases in some degree analogous	247
The pathology	251
The treatment	260

CHAPTER IV.

OF EPILEPTIFORM CONVULSION.

The history of epileptiform convulsion	268
In chronic softening of the brain	268

CONTENTS.

	PAGE
In chronic meningitis	271
In tumour of the brain	274
In induration of the brain	279
In atrophy of the brain	281
In congestion of the brain	281
In apoplexy	283
In inflammation of the brain	288
In fever	295
In urinæmia, &c.	297
In difficult dentition, worms, &c.	299
In the moribund state	303
The pathology of epileptiform convulsion	305
The treatment of epileptiform convulsion	326

CHAPTER IV.
OF SPASM . 346

The history of spasm	346
In catalepsy	346
In tetanus	347
In cholera	350
In hydrophobia	350
In ergotism	353
In cerebral paralysis	354
In certain diseases of the spinal cord	356
In certain cases of minor moment	360
The pathology of spasm	366
The treatment	380

PRELIMINARY CONSIDERATIONS

RESPECTING THE

PHYSIOLOGY OF MUSCULAR MOTION.

THE PHYSIOLOGY
OF
MUSCULAR MOTION.

SEVEN years have now elapsed since I first endeavoured to show[1] *that muscle contracts, not because it is stimulated to contract by nervous influence, or electricity, or any other so-called stimulus of contraction, but because something has been withdrawn from the muscle which previously prevented the free action of common molecular attraction.* The argument used at that time was partly physiological and partly pathological; in its best part it was so defective that I can now look back upon it with no feeling of satisfaction; but such as it was, it seemed to show, not only that this view of muscular action was consistent with actual facts, but that it furnished a means of arriving at the physical explanation of three of the most important problems in physiology— of muscular contraction itself, of the rhythmic action of the heart, and of certain independent

---

[1] 'The Philosophy of Vital Motion,' 8vo, London, Churchill, January, 1851.

movements of the vessels which are of fundamental importance in carrying on the circulation.

Four years later I returned to the subject,[1] and giving more prominence to its pathological bearings, I endeavoured to show that epilepsy and all other disorders in which muscular contraction is in excess, are only intelligible when they are interpreted by such a theory of muscular motion.

All this time, and until a very recent period, I was not aware that the thoughts of any other person had been led in the same direction, but I now find that a similar idea had been entertained by Professor Matteucci, of Pisa, and by Professor Engel, of Zurich—at least, so far as concerns the action of nervous influence in muscular motion.

Professor Matteucci's speculations upon the operation of nervous influence in muscular action, were communicated to the *Académie des Sciences* of Paris, in 1847[2]. Speaking of the nervous *fluid*, he says, " ce fluide développé, principalement dans les muscles, s'y répand, et, doué d'une force répulsive entre ses parties, comme le fluide électrique, il tient les éléments de la fibre musculaire, dans un état de répulsion analogue à celui présenté par les corps éléctrises. Quand ce fluide nerveux cesse d'être libre

[1] 'Epilepsy, and other disorders of the Nervous System which are marked by Tremor, Convulsion, or Spasm; their Pathology and Treatment,' 8vo, London, Churchill, 1854.

[2] 'Comptes Rendus,' March 17th, 1847.

dans le muscle, les éléments de la fibre musculaire s'attirent entre eux, comme on le voit arriver dans la roideur cadavérique.... Suivant la quantité de ce fluide qui cesse d'être libre dans le muscle, la contraction est plus ou moins forte." Professor Matteucci appears to have framed this hypothesis partly in consequence of certain considerations which seemed to show that the phenomenon of "induced contraction" was owing to the *discharge* of electricity in the muscle in which the "inducing contraction" was manifested—an idea originating with M. Becquerel—and, partly, in consequence of the analogy which he himself had found to exist between the law of contraction in muscle, and the law of the discharge in electrical fishes; but he does not appear to have attached much weight to the idea even as an hypothesis. Indeed, his own comment at the time is,—" j'ai presque honte d'avoir eu la hardiesse de communiquer à l'Académie des idées si vagues, et apparemment si peu fondées, et contre lesquelles on pourrait faire bien des objections, mais je pense que, parmi les théories physiques les mieux fondées aujourd'hui, il en existe qui ont débuté de cette manière, et il est certain que des hypothèses, aussi peu fondées que celles-ci, ont quelquefois pu produire ensuite des découvertes remarquables."

The views of Professor Engel upon the operation of nervous influence in muscular action are stated in these words. " So hat der Nerve die Aufgabe, nicht die Zusammenziehungen des Muskels zu veranlassen, sondern den Zusammenziehungen bis auf einen geringen Grad entgegenzuwirken. Im lebenden Organismus, in welchem Ruhe etwas Unmögliches ist, ist auch ein ruhender Muskel eben so wohl wie ein ruhender Nerv undenkbar, der Muskel in seinem beständigen Streben, sich zusammenzuziehen, wird vom Nerven daran verhindert, im Nerven macht sich das fortwährende Streben kund, die Zusammenziehung des Muskels auf ein gerechtes Mass zurückzuführen; das Ergebniss dieser zwei einander entgegengesetzen Eigenschaften des Nervens und des Muskels ist das, was man gemeinhin Zustand des Ruhe, Zustand des Gleichgewichtes, oder an Muskeln auch Tonicität nennt. Das Verlassen dieses Gleichgewichts ist die Bewegung einerseits, die Lähmung andererseits. Die Bewegung wird aber erzeugt, indem entweder der Einfluss des Nervens auf den Muskel herabgesetz wird, oder indem die Contractionskraft des Muskels unmittelbar gesteigert wird. Lähmung des Muskels fiudet sich gleichfalls entweder durch unmittelbare Vernichtung der Contractionskraft des Muskels oder durch eine übermässig gesteigerte Ein-

[1] "Ueber Muskelreizbarkeit." 'Zeitschrift der Kais, Köu. Gesellsch. des Aerlze zu Wien,' 1849.

wirkung des motorischen Nervens auf den Muskel. Sollen daher abwechselnde Muskelcontractionen zu Stande kommen, so ist die Gegenwart des lebendigen Nervens im Muskel unerlässlich, und auch bei unmittelbaren Muskelreizen können abwechselnde Zusammenziehungen nur erfolgen, so lange noch die Nerven lebensfähig sind; hört letzeres auf, so zieht sich der Muskel ohne Hinderniss zusammen. Diesen Zustand nennen wir die Todtenstarre." The reasons upon which these views are based would appear to be three in number. The first is to be found in certain facts, many of them very remarkable, which seem to show that the muscles of frogs become more apt to contract under mechanical irritation when they are abstracted from the main sources of nervous influence—as by removing the great nervous centres altogether, or by allowing time for the activity of these centres to become exhausted. The second depends upon the fact that the permanent contraction of *rigor mortis* is the state which supervenes when all signs of nervous influence are completely extinguished. The third is to be found in the fact that cramps and other forms of excessive muscular contraction are often seen to happen spontaneously in paralysed parts.

Later still—later than the time when I published my own views on the subject of muscular action,—I also find that Professor Stannius, of Rostock, refleeting upon the way in which *rigor mortis* is seen to be relaxed by blood,[1] has been led to a similar conclusion respecting the action of nervous influence upon muscle. Reflecting upon this fact, this physiologist considers—" dass es eine wesentliche Aufgabe der sogenannten motorischen oder Muskelnerven sei, die natürliche Elasticitäts grosse der Muskelfasern herabzusetzen und ihre Elasticität vollkommener zu machen; dass anscheinende Ruhe des Muskels, zum Beispiele, während des Schlafes, das Stadium solchen regen, den Muskel zu seinen Aufgaben weider befähigenden Nerveneinflusses anzeige; dass active Muskelzusammenziehung einen geregelten und begrenzten momentanen Nachlass des Nerveneinflusses auf den Muskel bezeichne; dass endlich die Nachweisung einer Muskelreizbarkeit, in der üblichen Auffassungsweise, ein durchaus vergebliches Bemühen sei." And afterwards he adds, " Ich muss es mir vorbehalten, später den Beweis zu führen, das diesse Anschauungsweise, so paradox sie immer auf den ersten Anblick sich anlassen mag, mit unserem thatsächlichen Wissen über Nerven und Muskelthätigkeit keineswegs im Widerspruch steht."

— I do not stand alone, then, in thinking that a great change is demanded in the theory of mus-

---

[1] 'Untersuchungen über Leistungsfähigkeit der Muskeln und Todtenstarre; Vierordt's Archiv für Physiol. Heilkunde,' Stuttgart, 1852.

cular action—a change which amounts to no less than a complete revolution—and hence I am encouraged to take up the subject anew, and point out the numerous particulars in which subsequent inquiry has shown that the old argument requires to be modified and expanded before it can hope to demand the attention of physiologists and pathologists.

In the present instance, I propose to confine myself, simply and exclusively, to the *Physiology of Muscular Motion*, and, leaving the pathology for the body of this work, I shall endeavour to establish the three following propositions:

I. That muscular contraction is *not* produced by the stimulation[1] of any property of contractility belonging to muscle.

2. That muscular elongation[2] is produced by the simple physical action of certain agents, electricity and others, and that muscular contraction is the simple physical consequence of the cessation of this action.

[1] The recognised opinion is that muscle is endowed with a vital property of contractility, and that muscular contraction is brought about when this property is called into action by certain agents, such as electricity or nervous influence. It is supposed, indeed, that this vital property of contractility is roused or excited or *stimulated* into a state of action when the muscle contracts, and hence the agents which thus rouse or excite or stimulate are called *stimuli*.

[2] The term *elongation* is used in preference to the term *relaxation* for reasons which will appear in the sequel.

3. That the special muscular movements which are concerned in carrying on the circulation—the rhythm of the heart, and the movements of the vessels which are independent of the heart—are susceptible of a physical explanation when they are interpreted upon this view of muscular action.

I. THE FIRST PROPOSITION.

THAT MUSCULAR CONTRACTION IS NOT PRODUCED BY THE STIMULATION OF ANY PROPERTY OF CONTRACTILITY BELONGING TO MUSCLE.

1. *That muscular contraction is not produced by the stimulation of electricity.*

In order to understand the mode in which muscle is affected by *electricity*, it is necessary to know something of those electrical actions of which living muscle, in common with several other living structures, is the subject.

It is no new idea that muscle is the subject of electrical actions. Thus, Galvani explained the contractions which arise in a recently killed and prepared frog, when its nerves and muscles are connected by a conducting arc—" arco conduttore "—by supposing that *animal electricity* had been *discharged* by the arc. Soon, however, the discovery of Volta, that electricity was produced by the contact of dissimilar metals, gave rise to the idea that these contractions were due, not to the discharge of animal electricity, but to the passage of a weak current from the arc itself; and this opinion continued to gain ground, until Humboldt gave additional weight to the claims of animal electricity, by showing that similar contractions were produced when the muscles and nerves of the frog were connected by a piece of recent nerve. A little later, and animal electricity was once more thrown into the shade by the discovery of the voltaic battery. Then followed a long period of forgetfulness, only broken by Nobili's discovery of the "current of the frog," and not terminated until Professor Matteucci took up the subject and demonstrated most conclusively the existence of electrical currents in several tissues, and in muscles among the rest. It is to Dr. du Bois-Reymond,[1] however, that belongs the honour of having investigated most successfully the difficult subject of animal electricity, and there is no better course open to us than to follow in the track which he has opened out.

In his investigations upon the "muscular current" (to use the term which Professor Matteucci has applied to the current of animal electricity developed in living muscle), Dr. du Bois-Reymond made use of a galvanometer, the general arrangement of which is very similar to the sinus-galvanometer of Poggendorff. In the first instance, he used an instrument, the coil of which consisted of 3,280 feet of wire, and with this he also discovered the "nerve current," of which more will be said presently; but subsequently he used a far more

[1] 'Untersuchungen über thierische Electricität,' Berlin, 1848.

sensitive instrument, of which some particulars must be mentioned.

In this instrument, the frame upon which the wire is coiled, the arch from which the needles are suspended, and the screws for receiving the ends of the coil, are fixed on a circular plate which can be rotated upon a central axis. The sides of the frame are 4·6 inches long, 3·1 inches high, and 1·6 of an inch apart. The depth of the space in which the lower needle swings, is 0·1 of an inch. The copper wire forming the coil is 5584 yards, or 3·17 English miles in length, and about ·0055 of an inch in diameter. The number of coils is no less than 24,160. The needles are cylindrical with each end sharpened out into a long point. They are 1·5 of an inch in length, ·03 in diameter, and the weight of the two is 4 grains. They are connected by a thin piece of tortoise-shell, nearly 1·6 of an inch in length, and weighing not more than 0·9 of a grain. Away from the coil, the astatic system was adjusted so as to make a single vibration in 33 seconds.

Each end of the coil is connected with a peculiar electrode which requires to be described in order to make some of the following remarks intelligible.

This electrode consists of a horizontal arm, a pair of platinum plates, a glass trough containing a saturated solution of common salt, a cushion of blotting paper (of which the upper end is made to bend over the edge of the trough while the lower end is made to rest upon a ledge which projects inwardly from the wall of the

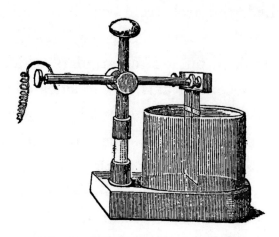

trough), a vertical pillar, and a wooden stand. The horizontal arm supports the platinum plates at one extremity, and at the other extremity it receives the wire of the galvanometer. The arm itself is moveable upon the pillar. The platinum plates are fixed to the arm by an appropriate clamp, and they hang so as to be immersed in the solution with which the trough is filled. Each plate is 2·5 inches in length, and 1 inch in breadth. Great care is taken in the preparation of these plates. It is absolutely necessary that they should be perfectly homogeneous (for any heterogeneity will give rise to currents when the circuit is closed), and in order to secure this they are cleansed successively with a mixture of alcohol and sulphuric ether, with nitro-muriatic acid, with distilled water, and last of all they are heated to incandescence for half a minute in the flame of a Berzelius' lamp. Great precautions are necessary, moreover, to preserve as well as to procure this homogeneity. A transitory current may be produced by the immersion of homogeneous plates, if the immersion of the plates of the two electrodes be not absolutely simultaneous; and to prevent this source of confusion, the plates of each electrode are kept continually immersed in the saline solution. A current might also arise from different conditions of different parts of the same plates if these plates were only partially immersed in the solution; and to obviate this difficulty, the parts above the solution are kept continually moistened by being wrapped in pieces of blotting paper of which the lower portion is immersed in the solution. Each electrode is furnished with two plates, partly to increase the surface by which any current may be able to enter the coil, and partly as an additional precaution against heterogeneity in the plates themselves,— for it is found that this cause of disturbance is less likely to operate when two plates are used than when only one plate is used. The cushion of blotting-paper is about 1·25 of an inch in breadth, and 2 inches in length, and when swelled out by absorbing the solution—about 0·5 of an inch in thickness. It is always soaked in the solution in which its lower portion is immersed; and its moist surface is therefore continuous with the surface of the solution. This cushion, indeed, is the real electrode, for it is through it that any current enters into or returns from the coil. The pillar which supports the horizontal arm and the parts attached to it, is insulated by a glass foot. Such is the electrode to which each end of the wire of the galvanometer is attached.

In completing the circuit, the cushions of the two electrodes may be placed in contact, or they may be connected by a third cushion, itself soaked in the same saturated solution of salt. When the instrument is not in use, the circuit is closed in this manner, and also (for additional security) by a piece of wire. Indeed, every precaution is taken to diminish the chances of any heterogeneity arising in the electrodes by making the circuit as complete as possible.

The galvanometer which I have used in repeating Dr. du Bois-Reymond's experiments, and for other experiments to which these have led me, was made[1] after

[1] This instrument, which is the first of its kind constructed in this country, was made by Mr. Becker, of Newman Street. Mr. Becker, moreover, entered with much spirit into the inquiries for which it was destined, and I derived very material assistance from his kind co-operation in some of the earlier experiments. Indeed, I shall always congratulate myself on the fact that I had recourse to his skilful assistance.

the pattern of the one which has been just described, or nearly so. The guage of the wire forming the coil in this instrument is number 38, or as nearly as possible that of the pattern coil, the weight of the wire entering into the coil 1 lb. 11 oz., the layers of the coil 154, the number of coilings 20,020. The coilings, therefore, are not quite so numerous as in the pattern coil—a difference owing in all probability to the silk winding around the wire being somewhat thicker; but the instrument to all appearance is not a whit less sensitive on this account. The needles were copied with as much exactness as possible, and the only difference in the astatic system is in the fact that the connecting piece is made of aluminium instead of tortoise-shell. The whole system was a little lighter—4·5 grains, instead of 4·9 grains. The degree of astaticism was such as to make the needles arrange themselves at right angles to the magnetic meridian, or thereabouts.

When in actual use, the galvanometer is placed upon a solid support where there will be as little vibration as possible, insulating pieces of glass are placed under the adjusting screws, and the coil is arranged so as to be across the magnetic meridian, or nearly due east and west. The electrodes may be on the same support as the coil or upon an adjoining table. In performing an experiment, the intermediate cushion, and the connecting wire, are removed, and the circuit is completed by placing the muscle upon the cushions, after having first covered the parts upon which it will actually rest with a small fragment of pig's bladder well moistened with white of egg. The bladder is used to prevent the direct action of the saline solution upon the muscle—an action which may of itself be sufficient to produce contraction.

Dr. du Bois-Reymond has examined the muscular current in man, rabbits, guinea-pigs, and mice; in pigeons and sparrows; in tortoises, lizards, adders, slow-worms, frogs and toads, tadpoles and salamanders; in tench; in freshwater crabs, and in earthworms;—and always with the same result. The animal which he ordinarily used was the water frog (*rana esculenta*), and this animal is undoubtedly the best suited to the purpose; but it is not necessary to be at the trouble to obtain these frogs from the Continent, for every experiment may be performed upon the common land frog (*rana temporaria*) of this country, if the galvanometer be as sensitive as the one above described, and if the frog be full grown. Indeed, I have not only repeated all Dr. du Bois-Reymond's fundamental experiments upon the common frog, but I have obtained more marked results than were obtainable from certain specimens of the *rana esculenta* which I had procured from the neighbourhood of Hamburg.

The primary phenomena of the muscular current, may be studied in any muscle, but most conveniently, perhaps, in the *adductor magnus* of the frog—most conveniently, because in this muscle it is easy to bring the ends of the fibres, or the sides of the fibres into separate relation with the cushions of the galvanometer. If, then, this muscle be laid upon the cushions, the results are these:—

If the two ends of the muscles are so laid; thus—

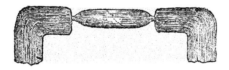

the needle of the instrument is deflected very slightly or not at all. In other words no sensible current is derived from the muscle. If the two sides of the muscle are placed in connexion with the cushions, the result is the same. But if the muscle be bent upon itself, and the cushions of the galvanometer so placed that one is in contact with the red flesh, and the other with the tendinous extremity; thus—

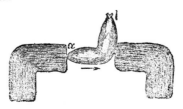

the needle of the galvanometer immediately gives evidence of a current in the direction of the arrow, that is, from the tendinous end. And, again, if the muscle be turned round so as to bring the other tendinous extremity to the cushion; thus—

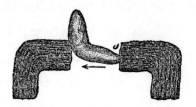

there is still a current, and this current still sets from the tendinous end. And thus it appears that the muscular current is not fixed in its course, in as much as it is made to set in the contrary direction when the muscle is turned round upon itself.

Similar results are also obtained by repeating these experiments after having first cut off the tendinous extremities of the muscle, for, on doing this, there is still no current, or a very feeble current, so long as the two ends only, or the two sides only, are in contact with the cushions; and there is a current, now somewhat stronger, which invariably sets from the end to the side, when the end of the muscle is placed in contact with one cushion, and the side with the other cushion.

On further examination, it is found that the different points of the longitudinal and transverse surfaces of a muscle, whether natural or artificial, possess electrical differences, and that these differences give rise to a current under certain circumstances. If, for example, two points of the longitudinal surface of the *adductor magnus*, which are equally distant from the middle of the length of the muscle, are placed upon the cushions of the galvanometer, there are no evidences of a current, or but very slight evidences; but if the two points are so chosen, that one is further from the middle than the other, thus—

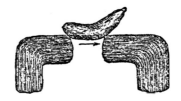

the needle shows the presence of a current from the point which is nearest to the end of the muscle. And so also with the transverse surface. There is no current if the two points in connection with the cushions are equally distant from the median point; and there is a current if one point be nearer to this point than the other. But when most decided, the current which is derived from different points of the longitudinal or transverse surfaces is very weak when compared with the current which passes between the longitudinal and transverse surfaces.

In order to explain these phenomena more clearly, Dr. du Bois-Reymond has constructed an

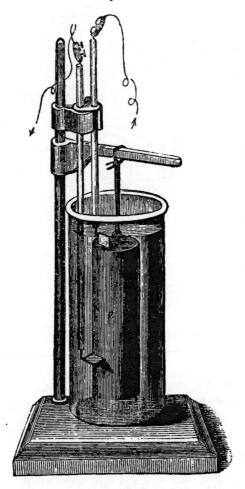

apparatus in which they are all reproduced, and by which it is possible to attain to a very exact idea respecting them.

One of these instruments, and this the most satisfactory, consists of three parts—an electro-motive cylinder, a glass vessel containing water, and an appropriate stand. The electro-motive cylinder is copper, covered with a coating of amalgamated zinc, except at the two ends. It is 6·1 inches high and 2·1 inches in diameter. The vessel for containing this cylinder is 3·5 inches in diameter, and sufficiently high to allow the electro-motive element to be fully immersed in it. The stand consists of a wooden base, a vertical pillar, and two clamps— one for supporting the cylinder and the other for carrying the two wires by which the current is carried from the cylinder to the galvanometer. The stand is simply a square piece of wood upon which the glass vessel rests, and from which the pillar rises. The pillar is a metal rod upon which the two clamps may be made to slide up or down. One of the clamps, a well varnished piece of brass, projects horizontally, and to it the electro-motive cylinder is tied by a piece of string; the other clamp carries a cork which is perforated, so as to carry the conducting wires. The wires themselves are terminated at their lower extremities by small pieces of platinum (0·6 of an inch), and, in order to insulate them more effectually, they are enclosed for some distance in portions of glass tubing, of which the lower extremity is hermetically sealed upon them. These tubes and the contained wires may be pushed up and down, and moved about, so as to allow the platinum ends to be applied to different parts of the electro-motive cylinder.

On connecting the upper ends of the conducting wires with the galvanometer, the needle is acted upon or not acted upon according to the position of the platinum ends upon the electromotive cylinder. If one end be placed upon the zinc surface and the other upon the copper extremity, as in the figure, the needle immediately diverges to the extent of from 15° to 20° degrees. If both ends are placed upon the zinc surface at an equal distance from the two extremities of the cylinder, where consequently the electric tension arising from the reaction of the zinc and copper at these extremities is equal, there is no current; but if the ends be drawn upwards or pushed downwards, a current begins to be manifested as soon as their relations to the extremities of the cylinder begin to be unequal, — a current which may move the needle from 5° to 10°. There is no current, also, when the two ends are placed so as to be equidistant from the middle of the extremity of the cylinder, and there is a current when they are moved, so as to be unequally distant from this point. In a word, all the electrical phenomena of a muscle of which mention has yet been made, are fairly represented in this apparatus.

— But there are other phenomena of the muscular current, some of great interest, which have yet to be noticed.

In the *gastrocnemius* of a frog, for instance, the muscular current does not return to the sides of the fibres from both ends of the fibres, or from each end indifferently, as it did in the *adductor magnus*, but it returns from *one* end, and however the muscle be turned about on the cushions (except for a short time before its final extinction), the current always passes in an *upward* direction from the tendo Achillis to the head of the muscle. There is also an upward current in the *extensor cruris* of the thigh, and in several other muscles. In some muscles, on the contrary, there is a current in a contrary direction. It is so also with that general current which is derived from large groups of muscles; thus the general current of a limb has an *upward* direction in the leg of a frog, and a *downward* direction in the arm of a man, while in the pigeon the direction is *downwards* in the thigh, and *upwards* in the leg.

Now in order to explain these differences it is necessary to follow Dr. du Bois-Reymond a little further, and study the electrical condition of the tendon and the manner in which this condition may react upon the muscular current—a not very difficult task.

Tendon, like proper muscular fibre, is found to be the seat of evident electrical currents. If, for example, the tendon of a rabbit be so placed that its natural longitudinal surface is in connection with one cushion and the artificial transverse section with the other, the needle of the galvanometer is seen to move through a few degrees—seldom more than 5° and at most not more than 8°. It is also seen that this current moves in the same direction as the muscular current, *i.e.*, from the end to the side, that it readily becomes reversed, and that it dies out more slowly than the muscular current. If the tendo Achillis of a frog be examined, the results are the same, only here the evidences of the current are very indistinct; and similar results are also obtained when a portion of elastic tissue from the ligamentum nuchæ of a recently killed wether is put in connection with the galvanometer.

This current of the tendon is indeed feeble, but it is sufficiently active to react positively upon the muscular current, and this reaction will explain some of the difficulties with which we are at present concerned. It will explain, for instance, how it is that the muscular current in the gastrocnemius of the frog becomes reversed when the muscle has been subjected for some time to a freezing temperature. It is still Dr. du Bois-Reymond who has discovered the fact of this reversal, and supplied the explanation. He has found, indeed, that the previous *upward* current of the gastrocnemius is *brought back again*, although in greatly diminished force, when the tendinous expansion is removed by the knife or destroyed by chemical or other means, and at the same time he has proved that this bringing back is really due to the removal or destruction of the tendinous expansion, by showing that no such effect is brought about by cutting or otherwise destroying the sides of the proper muscular fibres of the muscle. In other words he has traced the feeble *downward* current of the frozen gastrocnemius to the tendon, and shown, not only that as this time the current of the tendon is contrary to that of the true muscle, but also that the muscular current may become so much enfeebled as to be overruled by the current of the tendon.

In the same way, also, we may in all probability explain why it is that a feeble *downward* current takes the place of the previous *upward* current of the hind limb of the frog (a fact I have repeatedly noticed), and passes for a short time before the final extinction of all electrical actions; and that this reversal happens equally when the previous upward current has been allowed to die out gradually, or when it has been suddenly exhausted by a series of alternating shocks from an induction coil; for if the current of the tendon comes into play when the muscular current has been weakened by cold, it may also be looked for in any case in which the muscular current has become sufficiently weakened.

If, then, this be the effect of the tendon, it follows, almost as a necessary consequence, that the course of the muscular current in particular muscles will be affected by the arrangement of tendon belonging to the muscle, and that the muscular current, *cæteris paribus*, will escape from that end of the muscular fibre at which it encounters least resistance from the current of the tendon. And as the arrangement of tendon is different in different muscles, or even in the same muscle in different animals, it may be inferred that the course of the current will be different in different muscles, or in groups of muscles,—for the general current which is derived from groups of muscles, as from the muscles of a limb, is only the resultant of the current of the individual muscles, or rather, it is only the resultant of the currents of the individual muscular fibres, for evidences of a current obeying the same law are found in the smallest as well as in the largest portions of muscular tissue.

— It would also seem as if the muscular current were *weakened* during ordinary contraction; indeed, there can be no reasonable doubt that this is the case. In demonstrating this very important fact, Dr. du Bois-Reymond makes use of the gastrocnemius of a frog with a long portion of its nerve attached. This muscle is placed upon the cushions of the galvanometer, and the nerve is arranged in such a manner that a series of shocks from an induction coil can be passed through a portion of it. As soon

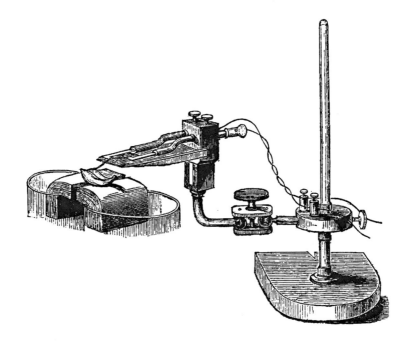

as the muscle is laid upon the cushions, the needle of the galvanometer is deflected to some distance from zero, and it continues to be deflected, though not to same extent, so long as the muscle remains in a state of rest; as soon as the muscle is tetanized by passing the interrupted current through a portion of the nerve, the needle immediately travels back again and oscillates on the other side of zero. These are the simple facts. As soon as the muscle is tetanized, that is to say, *the needle is acted upon by a reverse current.*

Now it cannot be supposed that this current is

due to the irruption of a current, from the induction apparatus by which the muscle is tetanized, into the circuit of the galvanometer, for both galvanometer and coil are carefully insulated. Moreover, there is the same reverse current (only in a less marked degree) when the muscle is tetanized by other means, as by subjecting the nerve to mechanical or chemical irritation, or by acting upon it by heat. Nay, the same current is seen to be produced by strychnine in a gastrocnemius which is still in living connexion with the nervous centres by means of the ischiatic nerve.

Nor is the reverse current, which is manifested during tetanus, to be regarded as a proof that there is a muscular current during contraction, whose direction is contrary to that of the current which plays during the state of rest. On the contrary, it is possible that the muscular current, before the state of tetanus was induced, may have given rise to a reverse current within the circuit of the galvanometer by evolving the secondary polarity of the platinum plates, and that this reverse current may be manifested during tetanus, in consequence of the proper muscular current having become *weakened*. And that this is the true explanation may be seen by the following modification of the same experiment.

The only difference between the experiment as

modified and the original experiment is this—that one of the electrodes, instead of being connected with the galvanometer by a continuous piece of wire, is connected by a broken wire, of which the two ends are made to dip into a small cup of mercury. The difference, that is to say, is in a simple contrivance for rapidly breaking or closing the circuit; for it must be plain that the circuit is broken when an end of the wire is raised out of the mercury, and closed when the same end is replaced in the mercury. In performing the modified experiment, the muscle is first laid upon the cushions, and a note made of the degree to which the needle of the galvanometer is deflected. Then the muscle is removed from the circuit of the galvanometer, and the instrument depolarized by raising one end of the wire out of the mercury. In the next place, the muscle is tetanized, and while it is in this state it is included in the circuit of the galvanometer by replacing the end of the wire in the mercury. In this way then, the current of the tetanized muscle is for an instant separated from that reverse current of secondary polarity, which is caused by the continued action of any current upon the instrument, and the result is that the needle travels in the *same* direction as that in which it travels under the current of the untetanized muscle, *but not to the same distance from zero*. In other words, the muscular current of the tetanized muscle is found to be *weakened,* but not changed—as it would appear to be if no care be taken to eliminate the influence of secondary polarity from the experiment. In several instances in which I repeated this experiment upon the ordinary frog, the primary deflection of the needle, under the current of the elongated muscle, was from 40° to 60°, and the permanent deflection from 5° to 7°, whereas the primary deflection of the needle, under the current of the tetanized muscle, was from 8° to 15°, and the permanent deflection from 1° to 2°.

Dr. du Bois-Reymond, however, is of opinion that it is not enough to look at the needle of the galvanometer in deciding this question, and he is of this opinion because the phenomenon of *induced* contraction (which phenomenon is manifested, as Professor Matteucci was the first to show, by placing the nerve of a second muscle upon a muscle in which contraction is to be brought about) appears to point to some *oscillation* in the current of the primarily contracting muscle, which oscillation is not revealed by the needle of the galvanometer. He is of this opinion, because the phenomenon of *induced* contraction, in being oscillatory and not continuous, appears to point to some oscillation in the current of the muscle in which the *inducing* contraction is manifested. Dr. du Bois-Reymond supposes further that the induced contraction is due to these *oscillations* in the muscular current of the muscle in which the *inducing* contraction is manifested; and supposing this, his next inference is that there could be no contraction in the muscle in which the *inducing* contraction is manifested unless its current had taken upon itself a similar oscillatory movement. Arguing from this phenomenon of induced contraction, he thinks, indeed, that the condition of the muscular current in muscular contraction is one of *oscillation* and not of simple *failure* (as the needle of the galvanometer would seem to show); and he concludes that there could be no contraction if the current remained *constant*. But it is not easy to perceive the force of this mode of reasoning. It is easy to understand that the needle of the galvanometer may be too sluggish to oscillate with every single oscillation of the current, but it is not easy to allow that the needle is too sluggish to take up a position in the mean of oscillation. And if the needle is not too sluggish for this, then the muscular current must be *weakened* if the current fails to keep the needle at the same degree of divergence as that at which it stood before the muscle began to contract,—for certainly the fact of trembling does not alter the fact of weakness. At any rate, this theory of oscillation is not necessary to account for the phenomenon of induced contraction, and that it is not will be sufficiently obvious hereafter.

— And, lastly, it is found that all evidences of the muscular current have disappeared when the muscle has passed into the state of *rigor mortis*. It is found, indeed, that the muscular current is most active when the "irritability" of the muscle is most perfect, that it fails *pari passu* with this "irritability," and that it has died out altogether when the muscle has passed into the state of *rigor mortis*.

— On turning from these considerations to those which concern the action of the ordinary galvanic current upon muscle, it is to be expected that the existence of the muscular current is not to be ignored. And further, it is to be expected that certain reactions between the two currents will arise out of the particular course of the muscular current. It is no doubt true, as Dr. du Bois-Reymond represents, that the muscular current passes from the end or ends to the sides of the muscular fibre; but it is also true that this current must complete its circle and return to the point from which it started. It is certainly true that the muscular current cannot have reached the ends of the fibre without having first reached the interior of the fibre, and that it cannot have reached the interior without having first passed through the exterior of the fibre. In other words, it is certainly true that the muscular current, in passing from the sides to the ends of the fibre, must have reached the interior by passing in a more or less *transverse direction across the exterior parts of the fibre*. Now, if such be the course of the muscular current, it is evident, first of all, that there is no way of passing the galvanic current through a muscular fibre in which this current will not cross the course of the muscular current. The galvanic current, it is true, will not always cross to the same extent, and to a certain point it may coincide with the course of the muscular current, as it will do when it passes along the interior of the fibre in the direction in which the muscular current is predominant — when it passes, for example, in an *upward* direction through the gastrocnemius; but if it coincides with the muscular current in its course along the *interior* of the fibre, it must cross the muscular current in that part of its course where, in order to reach the interior, it passes more or less transversely through the *exterior* of the fibre. And if the two currents cross in this manner, then must they clash; and (to an equivalent degree) neutralize each other. In a word, it is not enough to regard the muscle as a simple conductor, through which the galvanic current has to pass and take

2 §

possession; but it is necessary to regard it as the seat of a current which must be overcome before the galvanic current can pass and gain possession. Nor it is not enough to say that the muscular current returns when the galvanic current is suspended. The muscular current does return at this time—of this there can be no doubt, but there is also another current which springs into existence at the same time, and this is the ordinary *reverse* current which arises out of the secondary polarity of some part of the circuit. Just, then, as the muscle could not be looked upon as a simple conductor at the moment when the primary galvanic current began to pass, so now, it cannot be looked upon as a simple conductor at the moment when the muscular current returns to the muscle,—for before the muscular current can regain possession of the muscle it must contend with and overcome the reverse current above mentioned. It is evident, indeed, that there will be a clashing and equivalent neutralization between the muscular current and the reverse galvanic current at the moment when the circuit is opened, which is in every respect similar to that clashing and neutralization which took place between the muscular and primary galvanic current at the moment when the circuit is closed; and hence a moment in which electrical action is neutralized —a *moment of inaction,* as it may be called—may be supposed to precede both the establishment of the galvanic current and the return of the muscular current.

— What, then, it now remains to ask, are the phenomena which attend upon the passage of the galvanic current through the muscle, and how are they to be accounted for? The principal fact is, that a muscle contracts when the circuit is closed, and when the circuit is opened, but not during the time that the current is passing through it. Thus, in an experiment of Professor Matteucci in which a galvanic current was passed through the pectoral muscle of a pigeon from which every visible trace of nervous tissue had been carefully removed, the muscle was found to contract at the moment the circuit was closed, and at the moment the circuit was opened, but not during the passage of the current, and this order was found to be altogether irrespective of the direction of the current. In this experiment it was also found that the contraction on opening the circuit was less marked than the contraction on closing the circuit, —that both contractions became progressively less and less marked until they ceased altogether,—and that one or both of the contractions might be revived for a short time after their extinction by increasing the strength of the current.

Now in seeking for the explanation of these

phenomena it is difficult, if not impossible, to find any reason for supposing that the contractions are due to any direct action of the current, natural or artificial. For what is the case? The case is that the muscle does *not* contract so long as the galvanic current continues to pass through it. The case is that the muscle does *not* contract so long as it is left to the undisturbed possession of the muscular current. But on the other hand there is no difficulty in connecting the contractions with that clashing and mutual neutralization of the muscular and artificial current, direct or reverse, of which mention has been made as attending upon the commencement and cessation of the passage of the artificial current through the muscle,—for if contraction is absent when the artificial or natural current is manifestly present, and if contraction is present when the artificial or natural current is manifestly absent, then there appears to be only one course open, and that is to connect the contraction with the *absence* of the current.

Upon this view, also, it is intelligible that the contractions should become less and less marked as the experiment proceeds, and that the contraction on opening the circuit should be less marked than the contraction on closing the circuit. Removed from the body, the muscle is found to yield fainter and still fainter indications of a current until these indications cease altogether, and hence it follows that the neutralizing reaction between the muscular current and the artificial current will fail more and more as the experiment proceeds,—will fail, because to diminish this current is evidently to diminish the amount of reciprocal neutralization,—and, so failing, that the contractions will become progressively less and less marked, for if the contraction is connected with the neutralization of electrical action in the muscle, the degree of the contraction must be directly proportionate to the degree of this neutralization. It is, also, intelligible that the contraction on opening the circuit should be less marked than the contraction on closing the circuit, for the lapse of time and the disturbing influence of the artificial current upon the electromotive elements of the muscle, will combine to weaken the muscular current—will combine, that is, to render the contraction on opening the circuit less marked than the contraction on closing the circuit, for—to repeat what has just been said—to weaken this current is to diminish those neutralizing reactions between the two currents, which, upon this view, are directly measured by the degree of the contraction.

Nay, it is in some degree possible, upon the same view, to explain the fact that the contractions should be reproducible, after they have once ceased, by increasing the strength of the artificial current; for in order to explain this difficulty, it is only necessary to suppose—and the supposition is certainly allowable—that the weaker current had only penetrated the muscle superficially, and that the stronger current had penetrated more deeply and reacted with the current of muscular fibres which had been beyond the range of the weaker artificial current. This supposition is certainly allowable, for current electricity, although of very low tension, must yet possess some tension, and on that account it must agree in some degree with electricity of tension in preferring to occupy the surface of the body which serves as a conductor.

— There is, no doubt, much that is not altogether satisfactory in some of these speculations, and it cannot well be otherwise until a clearer knowledge of electricity is brought to bear upon the subject; but at the same time it must be evident that there is no reason for believing that muscle is stimulated into the state of contraction by electricity, and that this state of contraction passes off when this stimulation is at an end; and it may also be allowed that there is some reason for concluding that muscular elongation, and not muscular contraction, is the state which is produced by the action of electricity upon the muscle.

— Nor is there any objection to this view in the physical condition of the contracted and uncontracted muscle. At first sight, indeed, it would appear as if a stimulus had ceased to act when the muscle passes out of the contracted state, and it is no easy matter to get rid of this idea; but Professor Ed. Weber has shown, not only that the hardness of muscle in a state of contraction is simply owing to the straining of the muscle upon its attachments, but also that the contracted muscle is even softer than the uncontracted muscle when it is cut loose from these attachments. In other words, he has shown that the condition of the uncontracted muscle may be more correctly represented by the term *elongation* than by the term *relaxation*,—and hence the mere physical condition of the muscle does not oppose any objection to the idea that muscular elongation, and not muscular contraction, is produced by the action of electricity upon muscle.

2. *That muscular contraction is not produced by the stimulation of " nervous influence."*

" Nervous influence" is a convenient term, which includes more agencies than one. It includes certain agencies which are thought to be vital, and it includes other agencies which come within the scope of physical inquiry. It is not necessary, however, to endeavour to determine how much is vital, and how much is physical, for if one thing is more probable than another, it is that there is one common force underlying all agents, vital and physical, and that the differences of agency are owing, not to differences of force, but simply to the differences of circumstance in which one and the same force is manifested. Now of the several agencies included in the term "nervous influence," electricity is the one which is most easily investigated, and hence we will begin to interpret the mode in which muscle is affected by "nervous influence" from an electrical point of view.

Dr. du Bois-Reymond was the first to demonstrate the existence of actual electrical currents in nerves, and his demonstration is so masterly and complete as to leave very little to be done by others. The original discovery of these currents was made by means of the smaller galvanometer, which had been used in investigating the "muscular current," and the subsequent investigations were made, partly with this instrument and partly with his large instrument. The experiments are, in many respects, similar to the experiments upon muscle, and the results are strictly analogous.

Placing a piece of the ischiatic nerve upon the cushions, so that it touched one cushion with the artificial transverse section, and the other with the natural longitudinal surface, thus—

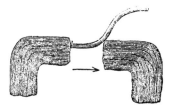

the needle of the galvanometer reveals the presence of a current from the end to the side of the nerve. Reversing the position of the nerve so that the other end is brought in contact with a cushion, thus—

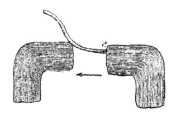

the current still sets from the end to the side of the nerve. But if the nerve be placed so that the two ends or the two sides are in contact, one end or one side with each cushion, there is no current. Moreover, if two points at equal distance from the middle of the nerve are placed upon the cushions, there is no evidence of a current; but, if one point is nearer to the middle than the other, then there are signs of a current which passes from the end towards the middle. Indeed, these phenomena of the " nerve-current," as this current has been called, are precisely similar to the phenomena of the "muscular current," with this exception—an exception arising in all probability from the smallness of the parts—that no evidence of a current could be found between dissimilar points in the transverse section of the nerve. It is found, also, that the same phenomena may be observed in purely motor and sensory nerves, as well as in mixed nerves, like the ischiatic.

Dr. du Bois-Reymond has also shown that a current sets from both ends when both ends were brought together by doubling the piece of the nerve into a loop, thus—

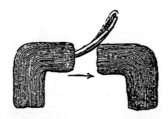

In the undisturbed condition of the nerve, however, as in the undisturbed state of the muscle, the nerve current is found to set in a particular direction, which, under ordinary circumstances, appears to be constant. Thus I find the nerve-current of the sciatic nerve to be in the same direction as that of the general current of the limb—that is, from the toes upwards, in the ischiatic nerve of all the animals I have examined, viz., the water-frog and land-frog, the mouse and rabbit. This may be easily seen in the frog, by laying the nerve of a galvanoscopic limb across the cushions, or by the more cruel expedient of bringing the same nerve into the same relations while it retains its connection with the nervous centres.

Like the muscular current in this respect, also, the nerve current dies out *pari passu* with the "irritability," and the extinction is complete when the "irritability" has departed. It dies out at about the same rate as the muscular current, and the only peculiarity is, that the act of death does not appear to be preceded by any reversal of the current. There is such a reversal if the nerve current be examined in a nerve which retains its connection with the muscle, and this equally whether the irritability has been allowed to die out gradually or whether it has been suddenly exhausted by a series of alternating shocks from an induction coil; but I find that this reversal is in some way connected with the reversal of the muscular current, for it ceases when the nerve is removed from the muscle, and it is never manifested when the nerve-current is investigated from the beginning in a separated nerve.

Dr. du Bois-Reymond has also shown that the "nerve current" agrees with the "muscular current" in that it affords evidence of enfeeblement *during muscular contraction*.

A frog is fastened upon a suitable frame, and then, after tying its common iliac artery, the ischiatic nerve is cut low down in the ham and

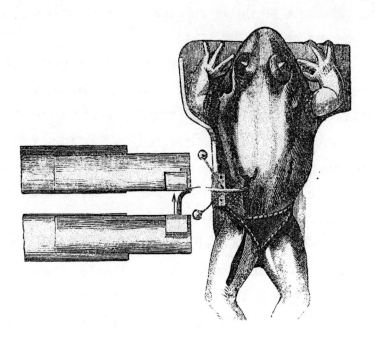

dissected out up to the vertebral column. After this the lower end of the nerve is bridged over the cushions of the galvanometer, so as to touch one cushion with its end and the other cushion with its side, and a note is taken of the degree to which the needle of the galvanometer is deflected by the "nerve current." The animal is then poisoned with two or three drops of a solution of nitrate of strychnia, and the effect of the tetanus upon the "nerve current" is attended to by watching the movements of the needle of the galvanometer. The experiment is simple and the result unmistakeable, for when the tetanus occurs *the needle recedes three or four degrees nearer to zero*, and this not only during the principal attacks, but also during those single shocks which are produced on touching the animal. It is seen further that the needle continues at this point so long as the tetanus continues, and that it again diverges from zero when the spasm passes off. It is seen, indeed, that the "nerve current" is enfeebled during muscular contraction. In some frogs upon which I repeated this beautiful experiment, the primary deflection of the needle under the nerve current *before* the supervention of the tetanic symptoms was from 15° to 20°, and the permanent deflection from 2° to 4°; and, *after* the supervention of these symptoms, the primary deflection was from 3° to 4°, and the permanent deflection scarcely perceptible. In these experiments I took the nerve from the cushions after testing its natural current, and replaced it in the wound. I then poisoned the animal with the strychnia, and when the spasms were fully established, I replaced the nerve upon the cushions. I did this in order to remove the nerve as much as possible from the desiccating influence of the atmosphere—an influence which might have put an end to the nerve current if the nerve had been allowed to remain upon the cushions in the interval during which the strychnia was taking hold upon the system.

— In turning from these considerations respecting the nerve current to those which concern the mode in which muscles are acted upon by galvanic electricity *through the instrumentality of the nerves,* there is one remarkable fact which claims immediate attention, and this is—*that the same results are produced by passing the current through a portion of a nerve as are produced by passing the current through the whole length of the nerve.* In the case of the galvanoscopic limb, for example, the same results are produced by including a small portion of the ischiatic nerve between the poles of the battery as are produced by placing one pole upon the extremity of the trunk of the nerve and the other upon the toes.

It is easily demonstrable, however, that the portion of the nerve which is not included between the poles of the battery is in the same electrical condition, or rather furnishes evidence of a current in the same direction, as the portion which is included between these poles, and hence it may merely be a natural consequence of the peculiar molecular structure of the nerve that the galvanic current cannot act upon a portion of a nerve without acting upon the whole nerve.

This is seen to be the case, by taking the sciatic

nerve of a frog, and arranging it so that a portion of it is included within the circuit of a properly insulated galvanometer, and another portion between the poles of a galvanic battery, also insulated. A galvanic current is then passed through the portion of the nerve which is included between the poles of the battery, and upon doing this *a current is found to pass in the same direction through the portion of the nerve which is included in the circuit of the galvanometer,*—if, that is, the galvanic current be sufficiently strong to overrule the " nerve current" when this current is contrary. If the galvanic current be very weak, and the " nerve current" be in a contrary direction, it may fail to set up a current in the same direction as its own in the portion of the nerve which is included in the circuit of the galvanometer, but if it fails to do this, it will not fail to *weaken* the " nerve current." Indeed, there is no exception to the statement here made—that the effect of passing a galvanic current of sufficient strength through any portion of a nerve, is to set up a current in the same direction in every part of the nerve.

Now, it cannot be that the galvanic current has spread directly into every part of the nerve, and thence into the circuit of the galvanometer, for the insulation of the galvanometer and battery requires that this current should be confined to that portion of the nerve which is included between the poles of the galvanic battery; and, therefore, it is necessary to suppose that the galvanic current has determined a corresponding arrangement in the electromotive elements of the nerve itself; but be the explanation what it may, the fact is undeniable, and there can be no doubt that a portion of a nerve cannot be acted upon by a galvanic current without a corresponding action being set up in other parts of the nerve.

What, then, it may now be asked, are the phenomena which are manifested in the muscles when a nerve, or a portion of a nerve, is acted upon by the galvanic current, and how are they to be accounted for?

When a nerve, or a portion of a nerve, is included in the circuit of a simple galvanic apparatus, the results, as seen in the muscles, are very remarkable. If the experiment be performed upon the nerve of a recently prepared frog's leg, the muscles of the limb are seen to contract when the circle is opened and closed, and to remain elongated so long as the current continues to pass; and, at first, no very marked differences in the degree of these two contractions are produced by changing the direction of the current. Afterwards, when the excitability of the nerve has become diminished, there begin to be certain differences in the degree of these contractions, which differences are determined by the direction of the current in the nerve,—the law being (1) that the contraction on opening the circuit is more marked than the contraction on closing the circuit, *when the current is said to be "inverse"*—when, that is, it passes from the expansion to the origin of the nerve; and (2), that the contraction on closing the circuit is more marked than the contraction on opening the circuit, *when the current is said to be "direct"*—when, that is, it passes from the origin to the expansion of the nerve. At a later stage of the experiment the contractions are found to become fainter and fainter, until they cease altogether, the rule being that the contraction which was most marked is continued for some time after the other has disappeared. In this experiment, the galvanic current may be passed in either direction, but not up and down the nerve alternately or indiscriminately, and this is a point of considerable importance. Indeed, on reversing the current it is found that the muscles will again begin to respond to the current, even after they have altogether ceased to respond to the former current. It is also found that the contractions which arise on reversing the current in this manner, will attend for some time upon the closure and disruption of the circuit; but not for so long a time as that during which they attended upon the previous current. It is even possible to reproduce the contractions more than once on reversing the current in this way, and some time may elapse before these remarkable alternations, or *voltaic alternatives* as they have been called, will come to an end. These peculiar alternations are to a certain extent independent of the direction of the current in the nerve, but at the same time the direction of the current has a very appreciable influence upon the results. If the current be *direct*—that is, from the origin of the nerve to its expansion, and if it be passed for some time continuously, and the circuit then opened and closed, the opening and closure of the circuit are not attended by any contractions in the muscular fibres; but if the current be *inverse*,—that is, from the expansion to the origin of the nerve, this is not the case, and provided the galvanic current be not too powerful, the current may be passed through the nerve for a much longer time than in the last instance, and the contractions may still attend upon the opening and closure of the circuit. Instead of exhausting the excitability of the nerve, as did the *direct* current, it would indeed seem as if the *inverse* current had augmented this excitability; and this was the opinion of Professor Matteucci, who first directed attention to these differences in the effects of the direct and inverse currents. At any rate, there is a *marked* contraction on opening the circuit after the *inverse* current has been passing for some time through the nerve.

Now, in explaining the action of the artificial current upon the nerve, as in explaining the action of the same current upon the muscular fibre, the key to every difficulty would appear to be in the recognition of certain reactions between the "nerve current" on the one hand, and the artificial current on the other hand; and all that is necessary is to use this key with sufficient carefulness.

At first sight, perhaps, it is difficult to understand how it is that the artificial current should act so differently according as it is passed up the nerve or down the nerve, but on referring to the particular reactions which must take place between the galvanic current and the nerve current under these circumstances, this difficulty is done away with. The irritability of the nerve is impaired or destroyed when the galvanic current through the nerve is *direct*—when it passes, that is, from the origin to the expansion of the nerve; and this is not to be wondered at if the irritability of the nerve is to be measured, as it assuredly is, by the activity of the "nerve current" in the nerve. For what is the case? The case is that the *direct* galvanic current has been passed in a direction which is contrary to the direction of the *current of the sciatic nerve* (*v.* p. 42), and that, having been so passed, it must especially tend to weaken or extinguish this current. On the other hand, the irritability of the nerve is augmented, or at any rate revived, when the direction of the galvanic current in the nerve is *inverse*, or when it passes from the expansion of the nerve to its origin. In other words, the irritability of the nerve is augmented or revived when the galvanic current is passed in the *same* direction as the *current of the sciatic nerve*. And thus it is in some degree intelligible that a property of the nerve, which is to some extent connected with the nerve current, should be impaired by what has been called (hastily perhaps) the *direct* current, and preserved by what has been called (not less hastily) the *inverse* current, for these results may after all be no more than the natural consequence of the way in which the galvanic and nerve currents clash in the one case and coincide in the other case.

On referring more particularly to the reactions which must take place between the artificial current and the nerve current, it is possible to understand why the muscles should contract only at the opening or closure of the circuit, and not during the passage of the current.

Now, it is very evident that certain difficulties would have to be removed before it can be held that the muscles contract because the galvanic current has acted upon the nerve in the sense of a "stimulus." It is indeed true that the muscles contract when the current begins to pass in the nerve and when it ceases to pass, but it is not less true that *the muscles do not contract during the actual passage of the current through the nerve.* It is also true that *the muscles will pass out of the tetanized state when a constant current is passed through the nerve.* Two facts are indeed certain— one long familiar to all physiologists, the other recently discovered by Dr. Eckardt[1]—which seem to show, if they show anything, that the *action* of the galvanic current upon the nerve is to produce elongation, and not contraction; for in the one case, a muscle *already elongated* is seen to remain *elongated* so long as the current continues to pass through the nerve; and in the other case, a *contracted muscle* is seen to *become elongated* when the nerve is acted upon by the current. And certainly there is no contrary conclusion to be drawn from the fact that the muscle contracts when the galvanic current begins to pass in the nerve, and when it ceases to pass.

When a nerve, or a portion of nerve, is included between the poles of a galvanic battery, it will be with the nerve current as it was with the muscular current when a portion of muscle was so included,—

[1] 'Grundzüge der Physiologie der Nervensystems,' Giessen, 1854.

for the nerve current and the muscular current are absolutely obedient to the same law. *When the circuit is closed,* the galvanic current will pass across the course of the nerve current, and so passing it will neutralize, and receive an equivalent amount of neutralization from, the nerve current. And thus an instant of neutralization, a moment of inaction, will precede the establishment of the galvanic current in the nerve. *When the circuit is opened,* the galvanic current will be suspended, and the nerve current will return to the nerve; but before the nerve current can thus return, it will have clashed for an instant with that *reverse* current which springs into momentary existence and traverses the nerve and other portions of the galvanic circuit upon the cessation of the primary galvanic current. In other words, the re-establishment of the nerve current after the cessation of the artificial current, will also be preceded by an interval of inaction, in which the first instalments of the nerve current and the momentary reverse current suffer that reciprocal neutralization which arises out of the differences of their direction. And hence it would appear that there is some neutralization of electrical action in the nerve at the moment of closing and at the moment of opening the circuit, and that the nerve is only under full electrical action either when the artificial current is passing through it, or when the nerve is left to the influence of its own current.

And if these neutralizing reactions between the galvanic current and the nerve current are connected with the contractions, it is possible to understand, in some measure, how it is that the contractions should vary as they are found to vary, at different stages of an experiment in which the nerve is acted upon by a galvanic current.

It is possible to explain why the contractions should gradually die out. In order to these contractions, the hypothesis assumes that the antagonism of the nerve-current is essential, and hence it follows that the contractions will die out *pari passu* with the current. Nor is it impossible to explain the particular and very singular mode in which the contractions die out.

When the *direct* current is passed through the sciatic nerve, *the contraction on breaking the circuit is the first to die out,* and so it should be according to the premises. Under these circumstances, indeed, the effect of the artificial current—which is *opposed* to the current of the sciatic nerve—is to weaken the nerve-current, and hence it follows that the nerve-current will be weaker when it returns to the nerve after the galvanic circuit is broken, than it was before the nerve was included in that circuit. Under these circumstances, indeed, the effect of the galvanic current will be to weaken the nerve current, and in that way to render that contraction less marked which happens when the galvanic current ceases to pass,—for this contraction, according to the premises, is proportionate to the amount of neutralization which takes place between the nerve current and the artificial current—in this particular case, the reverse current. And hence it is—as soon as this nerve current has become weakened by the action of the artificial current upon the nerve—that the apparent effect of the so-called *direct* galvanic current will be to weaken the contraction which happens when the circuit is broken more than to weaken the contraction which happens when the circuit is closed.

When, on the other hand, the so-called *inverse* current is passed through the sciatic nerve, *the contraction on closing the circuit is the first to die out,* and so it should be according to the premises. Under these circumstances, the artificial current is passed in the *same* direction as the current of the sciatic nerve, and its effect is to revive the nerve current rather than to exhaust it. Under these circumstances, indeed, the effect of the galvanic current is to revive the nerve current, and in that way to perpetuate the contraction which happens when the galvanic circuit is broken. And hence—as soon as the nerve current is really weakened by the action of the galvanic current upon the nerve—the apparent effect of the *inverse* current will be to weaken the contraction which happens when the circuit is closed more than the contraction which happens when the circuit is opened.

Nor is there anything unintelligible in the *voltaic alternatives* when the aid of the galvanometer is brought to their interpretation. For what is the simple fact? The fact is that the direction of the current in the sciatic nerve is altered by the prolonged passage of a galvanic current, and that *the nerve current has become reversed when the closure or opening of the galvanic circuit ceases to provoke contraction in the muscles supplied by the nerve.* This fact I have ascertained by repeated experiments upon the common frog. So long, indeed, as the muscles continue to contract when the galvanic circuit including the nerve is closed or broken, so long does the nerve current continue to pass in the same direction as at first; and when the contractions on opening or closing the circuit have come to an end, then the nerve current has become reversed. So long, moreover, as muscular contractions attend upon the opening or closure of the circuit after the galvanic current has been reversed, so long does the nerve current continue to be reversed also. In the common frog I have not been able to pursue the voltaic alternatives beyond the second stage, for it always happened that at the end of this stage the reversal of the galvanic current had no further effect in renewing the contractions. At this time, also, it always happened that the nerve current had become extremely faint or altogether undistinguishable. In a word, then, there is always the same antagonism of the nerve current and the artificial current at the moment of the contraction, and when the contraction has come to an end the change may be traced to the cessation of this antagonism. And thus, upon these principles, the voltaic alternatives cease to be altogether unintelligible.

— Looking at muscular action, then, in relation to the *electrical* changes of the nerves concerned in this action, it would seem that muscular elongation is coincident with the *action* of natural or artificial electricity upon the nerve, and that muscular contraction is connected in some way with the diminution or annihilation of this action; and no reason has yet arisen which can support the idea that any vital property of nerve has been called into active exercise during the time of contraction by the "stimulus" of electricity.

— And, certainly, there is little reason to believe that muscular contraction is produced by any stimulation derived from the nervous centres.

Indeed, there are certain facts which seem to be altogether fatal to such an opinion.

After destroying the spinal cord in the lumbar region of a pigeon, the muscles of the paralysed legs are soon found to become hard and contracted. At first these muscles are soft; in a few days they become somewhat hard; and, after a few weeks, they pass into an evident state of contraction—a state which serves to keep the legs continually extended and divergent. This fact was first noticed by Drs. Brown-Séquard[1] and Martin-Magron.

It has also been pointed out by the same physiologists that the facial muscles of a rabbit become contracted after the division of one of the facial nerves, and that not on the healthy side, as in man, but on the paralysed side. This deviation goes on gradually increasing for three or four weeks, and at last it may be very considerable. In one case, twenty-one months after the operation the bones even had become altered in form, and the whole face had a strong twist towards the paralysed side. In addition, also, to this permanent state of contraction, there is a marked disposition to tremor and convulsive movement in the paralysed muscles, particularly when the breathing of the animal is temporarily interfered with. In a dog, a cat, a

[1] 'Experimental Researches applied to Physiology and Pathology.' New York, 1853. By E. Brown-Séquard, M.D., p. 104.

guinea-pig, there was generally no permanent contraction on either side after division of the facial nerve, but convulsive movements were very common in the paralysed muscles. It is also evident that the nerve could have had no share in these movements, for its peripheric portion had entirely lost its vital properties upon the fifth day after the operation, or thereabouts.

There are also certain experiments by Dr. Brown-Séquard,[1] which show that the muscular power of the hind legs of a frog becomes greatly increased *after* the division of the spinal cord.

In these experiments weights of different sizes are suspended from a small hook that has been previously attached to one of the hind legs a little above the heel. The animal is then held up by its fore limbs, and a weight that is just sufficient to put the hind leg gently upon the stretch is placed upon the hook. In the next place the toe of the weighted leg is pinched, and the weight is changed for one heavier until the animal is no longer able to withdraw its leg from the torture to which it is subjected. This being done, the next thing is to divide the spinal cord immediately behind the second pair of nerves; and to go on testing the muscular power of the paralysed legs. The results are very strange. Immediately after the operation, the

[1] 'Comptes Rendus,' May 10th, 1847.

MUSCULAR MOTION.

the muscular power that can be put forth by the weighted leg when the toe is pinched is sometimes nil, but generally it is no more than a third or fourth of what it was before the operation. Fifteen minutes later this power is evidently rallying. In twenty or five-and-twenty minutes it has recovered all it had lost. An hour after the operation it is greater than it was before the operation, perhaps doubled. An hour or two later still it is certainly doubled, and possibly trebled; and from this time up to the twenty-fourth hour, when the increase generally attains its maximum, it goes on slowly augmenting. The particulars of two experiments with very fine frogs (A and B) were as follows, the weights raised being expressed in grammes:

	Before the Operation.	Immediately afterwards	5 minutes afterwards.	15 minutes afterwards.	25 minutes afterwards	1 hour afterwards	2 hours afterwards.	4 hours afterwards	24 hours afterwards.	48 hours afterwards.
A	60 gram.	20	45	60	80	130	140	140	150	150
B	60 gram.	10	30	40	60	100	120	130	140	140

When the increase of the muscular power has attained its maximum, it may remain nearly stationary for six, ten, fifteen, or twenty days, and after this time it fails by slow degrees. In a month, if the animal lives, this power will have fallen to its original value before the operation; and at the expiration of six, seven, or eight months, it may have fallen still lower, until it is not more than a third or a half of this value. It is possible, however, that the increased muscular power would not have failed in this way if care had been taken to exercise the paralysed limbs by galvanism.

Nor is it easy to agree with Dr. Marshall Hall in thinking that this increase of muscular power is due to an increased stimulation of the muscles on the part of the spinal cord (which inordinate stimulation had come into play because the controlling influence of the brain had been withdrawn), for there are other experiments which show plainly enough that the muscular power is augmented, not only in a similar but even in a higher degree, after the muscle has been cut off altogether from the spinal cord.

In the paper on muscular irritability, to which reference has already been made, and which is deserving of study, as well for the facts as for the opinions contained in it, Professor Engel, of Zurich, has shown that muscles are more prone to enter into the state of contraction after the complete removal of the cerebro-spinal system. In this experiment he clips out the whole of this system, bones and all, and, after five or ten minutes, he finds that the muscles have become so irritable as to be thrown into a state of contraction by a blow on the table. He finds, indeed, that the muscles are as irritable as they are in narcotized frogs.

Some very conclusive evidence to the same effect is also furnished in the following experiment by Dr. Brown-Séquard.[1] In this experiment the spinal cord of a frog is divided immediately behind the roots of the brachial nerves, and then the nerves proceeding to *one* of the hind legs are cut through at the points where they leave the cord. *Two hours later both the hind limbs are separated from the body,* and the contractility of their muscles is tested by the prick of a needle and by galvanism. This is the experiment. The result is *that the "irritability is augmented" in both these limbs, and that this augmentation is most considerable in the limb whose nerves had been divided—in the limb, that is to say, which had been cut off from the spinal cord.*

This result is entirely opposed to the conclusion which had been previously arrived at by Dr. Marshall Hall, but, as Dr. Brown-Séquard shows, this conclusion is not at all warranted by the experiment upon which it is based. Dr. Hall paralysed one of the hind legs of a frog, by dividing its nerves, and then tested the "irritability" of this

[1] Op. cit. p. 68.

limb—first, by passing a galvanic current through the animal, and afterwards, by poisoning with strychnia. In this way he produced contractions in the different muscles, and, as might be expected, he found that these contractions were less marked in the paralysed limb. But this experiment does not show that the paralysed muscles had lost any of their irritability. On the contrary, it only shows that they had been put almost altogether out of the field of action—for strychnia has scarcely any action, and galvanism has *comparatively* little action, upon muscles which are not in connexion with the nervous centres—and that they did not contract, simply because they had been thus put out of this field of action.

Now it is very difficult to reconcile these several facts with the idea that muscular contraction is produced by any stimulation derived from the nervous centres, and if any conclusion may be drawn from them it is one, or it would seem to be one, which must harmonize with that which has been already drawn from the electrical aspect of nervous influence.

— But, it may be asked, is not a fatal objection to this view to be drawn from the mode in which the will acts in producing muscular contraction? Is it not certain that the will acts in this case by stimulating the muscle to contract? It is difficult, no doubt, to think differently. It is more than difficult to wean the mind from so old an idea. But, on the other hand, it must not be forgotten that the will may have *acted* in bringing about muscular contraction, not by imparting anything to the muscles, but by withholding something from the muscles; and this being the case, we may well refuse to allow a mere opinion respecting the action of the will, however sanctioned by time that opinion may be, to rank as an objection to a view of the action of " nervous influence " in muscular motion, which view appears to arise necessarily out of the general history of "nervous influence" as concerned in muscular motion.

— And if this last objection may be set aside, then there appears to be no difficulty in assenting to the proposition at the beginning of this section, which is, *that muscular contraction is not produced by the stimulation of " nervous influence."*

3. *That muscular contraction is not produced by the stimulation of the blood.*

Arguing from the comparative anatomy of muscle, it would seem as if a muscle were not most disposed to contract when it is most liberally supplied with blood. It would even seem as if the degree as well as the duration of contraction were inversely related to the supply of blood: thus, this degree and duration of contraction is greater in the voluntary muscles of fishes and reptiles than in the voluntary muscles of mammals and birds; greater in involuntary than in voluntary muscles; and greater in the muscles of any given animal during the syncope of hybernation than during the fever of summer life.

The fact, moreover, that *rigor mortis* may be "relaxed," and the lost "irritability" restored to the muscle, by the injection of blood into the vessels—a fact which has been abundantly demonstrated by Dr. Brown-Séquard[1] and Professor Stannius[2]—would appear to be in direct contradiction to the idea that the muscle is in any way stimulated to contract by the blood.

Dr. Brown-Séquard placed a ligature around the aorta of several rabbits, immediately behind the origin of the renal arteries, and in a short time he found that the hind limbs were deprived of feeling and power of motion. He then waited until *rigor mortis*, or a rigidity like *rigor mortis*, had seized upon the paralysed parts, and when this state had lasted for about twenty minutes he untied the ligature, and found that the sensibility and power of motion

---

[1] 'Comptes Rendus,' 9 et 25 Juin, 1851.

[2] 'Archiv für Physiologische Heilkunde' (Vierordt's), Heft i, Stuttgart, 1852.

returned as the blood again made its way to the parts from which it had been excluded.

A still more conclusive experiment was performed upon the arm of a criminal who had been guillotined at 8 a.m. on the 12th of July, 1851. This arm, which was severed from the body, was in a state of perfect *rigor mortis* at 11 p.m.—fourteen hours after decapitation—and at this time the experiment was commenced by injecting a pound of defibrinated dog's blood into the brachial artery. As the blood began to penetrate into the vessels, some reddish spots appeared in different parts of the skin of the forearm, of the arm, and more particularly of the wrist. Then these spots became larger and larger, and the skin acquired the appearance it has in rubeola. Soon afterwards, the whole surface had a reddish-violet hue. A little later still, and the skin had acquired its natural living colour, elasticity, and softness, and the veins stood out distinct and full as during life. Then the muscles relaxed, first the fingers and lastly the muscles of the shoulders, and on examination they were found to have recovered their lost irritability. At 11·45 p.m. the muscles were more irritable than they had been at 5 p.m., at which time the corpse was first examined; and this degree of irritability was kept up, without abatement, until 4 a.m., when fatigue compelled Dr. Brown-Séquard for the time to abandon the experiment. When the experiment commenced the temperature of the blood was 73° Fahr., and that of the room 66° Fahr.

The subject of another experiment was a full-grown rabbit, which had been killed by hæmorrhage. Dr. Brown-Séquard waited until *rigor mortis* had fully set in, and then injected the defibrinated blood of the same animal into one of the hind limbs, which limb had been previously removed from the body. Fifteen minutes afterwards the muscles had lost their stiffness, and responded readily to mechanical or galvanic irritation. From this time, through the night, until 3 p.m. on the day following, the blood was injected at intervals of from twenty to thirty minutes, and all this time the muscles were perfectly soft and irritable. All this time, also, the muscles of the other hind limb, and of the rest of the body, were in a perfect state of *rigor mortis*. From 3 p.m. to 4·30 p.m. the injections were discontinued, and when they were resumed the limb had again become rigid, with the exception of a few bundles of fibres here and there. The effect of the injections was precisely as at first, and when they were again abandoned, from the lateness of the evening, the muscles were as soft and irritable as before. On the following morning, the limb upon which the injections had been practised was in a perfect state of cadaveric rigidity, while the muscles of the rest of the body, which had been left to themselves, were already beginning to pass out of this state. On the third morning the *rigor mortis* of the left limb was undiminished, and the other muscles of the body were in an advanced stage of putrefaction.

About the time that Dr. Brown-Séquard was engaged with these interesting experiments, Professor Stannius, without any knowledge of what was being done in Paris, was carrying out an analogous series of inquiries in Rostock. Dr. Brown-Séquard published the account of his experiments in June, 1851; Professor Stannius published his account in the beginning of 1852; and therefore the first-named physiologist has the priority in so far as their results agree.

The experiments of Professor Stannius were performed upon young dogs, and two will serve as examples of the fifteen which are given.

On the 21st of July, 1851, at 7·30 a.m., Dr. Stannius tied the abdominal aorta and crural arteries of a young dog. About 10·15 a.m. the muscles began to stiffen in the parts from which the blood was excluded, and at 10·45 a.m. both hinder extremities were stretched out, and perfectly stiff and cool. At 11·40 a.m. the ligatures were loosened, and the blood was seen and felt to penetrate into the empty vessels. At 11·45 a.m. both hinder extremities were warmer, and the right appeared to be a little more flexible than the other. At noon these limbs had recovered their flexibility, and it appeared once *as if the left had moved spontaneously,* but no sign of pain was caused by pinching the toes. At 12·25 a.m. incisions were made into both paralysed limbs, and everywhere the muscles were seen to contract upon the application of the electrodes. At one point, also, *there was evidence of pain,* for the animal, which was before quiet, gave a sudden plunge forwards. Death happened unexpectedly at 12·28 p.m.

A similar operation was performed upon another young dog, on the 22d of July, 1851, at breakfast time. At noon there were no evidences of stiffness in either of the hind limbs, but the muscles below the knee had ceased to respond to the touch of the electrodes. At 2·15 p.m. both these limbs were stretched out and rigid, and all evidences of irritability were at an end. At 2·35 p.m. the ligature around the aorta was untied, and at 2·50 p.m. the ligatures around the crural arteries. At 3·35 p.m. the application of the electrodes caused strong contraction in the muscles of both thighs, and weaker contractions in the muscles of the left leg below the knee, while at the same time nearly all traces of rigidity had disappeared from both limbs. At 5·35 p.m. every trace of stiffness had disappeared, and the muscles responded perfectly to the prick of a knife, as well as to the touch of the electrodes. On the following morning the animal was found dead, and the rigidity of death was fully established everywhere.

Now, the stiffness of which mention is here made is perfectly identical with *rigor mortis*, and this will appear from the following experiment. In this experiment, the aorta and crural arteries of a young whelp were all carefully tied, and the operation was over at 8·22 a.m. At noon all irritability had disappeared, and the muscles behind the ligature had become perfectly rigid. Seven and thirty hours after the operation the animal was still alive—at least in its anterior half—and upon the whole it was comparatively fresh and quiet. On the following morning it was found dead, with the parts *before* the ligature in a state of *rigor mortis*, and with the parts *behind* the ligature, not in a state of *rigor mortis*, but flaccid, moist, and partially putrescent. In other words, the parts *behind* the ligature were in the state which comes on after *rigor mortis*, and hence it follows that the stiffness which existed in these parts before the complete death of the animal must have been identical with *rigor mortis*.

Now, these experiments would only seem to be intelligible upon the supposition that the influence of the blood, be the *modus operandi* what it may, is exercised in counteracting, and not in causing, muscular contraction; and this conclusion, which I had drawn from the experiments of Dr. Brown-Séquard before my attention was directed to those of Dr. Stannius, is the same conclusion as that which (*v.* p. 6) Dr. Stannius himself has drawn from his own experiments.

— There are, however, certain facts[1] which seem to show that living, irritable, muscle is affected differently by arterial and by venous blood, and these facts have led Dr. Brown-Séquard to think that the office of arterial blood is to minister to the nutrition of muscular and other tissue, and to the storing up of contractile and other forms of power, and that the office of black blood—ordinary venous blood, or the blood of asphyxia—is to supply a stimulus by which the power derived from the red blood is called into action. Hence, according to this view, the function of venous blood is not a whit less important to the interests of the economy than that of arterial blood.

One argument in favour of the idea that muscle and other contractile tissues are stimulated to contract by venous blood, is based upon the well-known fact that these tissues are thrown into violent and general contraction when the whole mass of blood has become venous, as in asphyxia.

[1] Op. cit. and 'Comptes Rendus,' No. 16, 1857.

Another argument, also found among the phenomena of asphyxia, is derived from the fact that the left ventricle of the heart appears to pulsate more powerfully during the first moments of asphyxia, for at this time the pulse is fuller and firmer, and the mercury is raised to a higher point in the hæmadynometer.

Other arguments are based upon certain original experiments of Dr. Brown-Séquard.

In one of these experiments the abdomen of some mammiferous animal, generally a rabbit, was opened, and black or red blood was injected alternately into the aorta above the origin of the renal arteries. On injecting black blood convulsive movements were set up in all the parts to which the blood had penetrated; on injecting red blood these movements were suspended. The convulsions, moreover, were most violent when the blood was blackest, and most speedily brought to an end when the blood was richest in oxygen.

In another experiment the pregnant uterus of a bitch or doe-rabbit was separated from its connections with the cerebro-spinal centres, and blood was injected into the aorta. On injecting black blood the uterus was thrown into a state of contraction, and one or more fœtuses were expelled; on injecting red blood this contraction passed off.

Dr. Brown-Séquard says further, that muscles of

animal life, paralysed by the division of their nerves, behave in the same manner under the influence of red and black blood, with this difference only, that the contractions caused by the black blood are less marked than in the two experiments just mentioned.

Now these are facts which show unequivocally that muscle is affected very differently by venous blood and by arterial blood, but they are very far from showing that muscle is stimulated to contract by venous blood.

It may, indeed, be questioned whether the convulsions of asphyxia are not rather due to the want of the stimulus of red blood than to any stimulus derived from the black blood with which the system has become charged; for it is certainly true that the muscles are similarly convulsed when an animal is bled to death. In other words, it is certainly true that the muscles are similarly convulsed, as well when the animal is left without blood as when it is left full of venous blood.

Nor can it be allowed that the (apparently) more powerful contraction of the left ventricle during the first moments of asphyxia are due to increased stimulation on the part of the venous blood; for the fuller and firmer pulse, and the rise of the mercury in the hæmadynometer may be owing, not to increased contraction in the ventricle, but simply (as is indeed allowed on all hands) to the fact that there is some impediment to the free flow of blood through the capillaries of the systemic circulation—an impediment, that is to say, by which the systole of the ventricle is made to expend itself with greater force upon the coats of the intermediate arteries.

Again, it may be questioned whether the muscular contractions which are produced in the two other experiments, when black blood is injected into the vessels, may not also be due to the want of some stimulus belonging to the red blood rather than to the action of any stimulus derived from the venous blood. At any rate it is well known that the uterus has often contracted and expelled its contents when a pregnant animal has been bleeding to death. And there are several facts on record in which the human uterus, even, has expelled its burden after the mother has yielded to the utter syncope of actual death.

As it seems, however, the grand difficulty in the way of accepting this idea—that muscle is stimulated to contract by venous blood—is a chemical difficulty. For what is the main difference between arterial blood and venous blood? It is that the oxygen of the former has in the latter become displaced by carbonic acid. Now carbonic acid has an action upon all parts of the nervous system which minister to intelligence or sensibility—upon all parts of the frame indeed, with the supposed exception of those which minister to motion—which action is so obviously opposed to that of stimulation, that it is extremely difficult to suppose that carbonic acid can be a stimulus in any case. Indeed, it is so difficult, as to make it wellnigh impossible to entertain such a supposition for a single moment.

— Nor is there any reason to believe that any kind of blood is ever a stimulus to muscular contraction. It is possible, perhaps, that such an idea might be gathered from the fact that the convulsions of hæmorrhage and asphyxia come to an end when the bleeding or choking animal is upon the point of death; for looking at this fact in one point of view it may seem as if the convulsions had come to an end because the stimulus of arterial blood was taken away. At the same time a conclusion such as this is neither natural nor necessary. Thus: if it be asked how it is that the loss of blood, or the want of arterial blood, is attended by convulsion, the answer must be that the muscles are affected, not directly, but indirectly. A certain change, be this what it may, is produced in the nervous centres, and this change issues in convulsion, if the nerves discharge their office of conductors between the nervous centres and the muscles. This is evident in this one fact, that the convulsed state of a muscle is immediately put an end to by the division of its nerve. And this being the case, the question is as to the condition of the nerves at the time when the convulsions of hæmorrhage or asphyxia come to an end. Have the nerves at this time ceased to be conductors between the nervous centres on the one hand and the muscles on the other? Now it is certain that a fair supply of red blood is necessary to preserve the conducting power of the nerves. Thus, when the principal vessel of a limb is tied, the sense of touch and the power of movement are paralysed, and this state of paralysis continues until the collateral circulation is established. And if it be certain that a fair supply of red blood is necessary to preserve the conducting power of the nerves, then it is reasonable to suppose that the nerves may have ceased to conduct all natural telegraphic messages at the time when the convulsions of hæmorrhage or asphyxia come to an end, for at this time the supply of such blood to the nerves must be defective in the extreme. And if the nerves have ceased to be conductors the convulsions must cease, for in muscles which are isolated from the nervous centres, and left to themselves, the "muscular current" and the "nerve-current" will be re-established in the muscle, and as a consequence of this the contraction will disappear. And not only must the muscles become elongated under these circumstances, but, according to the same process of reasoning, they must continue elongated until they are allowed to pass into the state of *rigor mortis* by the dying out of the "muscular current" and "nerve current."

In this way, then, it appears to be possible to set aside the apparent objection which has been mooted, and hence the fact that an animal is convulsed by loss of blood or by want of arterial blood, becomes an indirect argument against the idea that muscle is roused into a state of contraction by the stimulation of the blood, while at the same time it corroborates in some degree what has been already said upon the relation of nervous influence to muscular contraction, inasmuch as the loss of blood or the want of arterial blood must necessitate a less active condition of the nervous centres, and (as consequent upon this less active condition) a less liberal supply of "nervous influence" to the muscles during the convulsions.

— In a word, there is no sufficient reason for supposing that muscle is ever excited to contraction by the stimulation of the blood, and there is some reason for believing that muscular elongation and not muscular contraction is coincident with this action.

4. *That muscular contraction is not produced by the stimulation of any mechanical agent.*

When a muscle is touched by a needle or any other mechanical agent the contraction which follows is referred to the stimulation of some vital power of contraction inherent in the muscle; but this conclusion may well be called in question after what has been said already. After what has been said, indeed, it would rather seem that the foreign body had served to *discharge* something of which electricity was one of the signs, and that the contraction was the result of this discharge. At the same time this idea is not without its difficulties.

The first difficulty is to be found in the fact that the muscle will contract with equal readiness and power whether it be insulated or not insulated, or whether it be touched with a conductor or a nonconductor. This is a difficulty, but it is one which may perhaps be overcome by interpreting the electrical history of the muscle by some points in the history of the electrical organs of the torpedo. Nor is this mode of interpretation at all illegitimate, for the analogy between the electrical organ and muscle has been abundantly proved by Professor Matteucci and others. Thus: the nerves of the electric organs arise from the anterior tract of the spinal cord, and terminate in loops or loop-like plexuses; and in this they agree with the nerves of the muscles. The electric organs are paralysed by the division of their nerves; and in this they agree with the muscles. The electric organs are made to discharge their fire by irritating the ends of the divided nerves which remain in connexion with them, and the discharge is limited to the part to which the irritated portion of the nerve is distributed; the muscles also contract under these circumstances, and the contraction is equally localized. The electric organs are exhausted by exercise and recruited by repose; so are the muscles. And, lastly, the action of strychnia upon the two organs is analogous, in that a state of tetanus is produced in the muscle, and a succession of involuntary discharges from the electric organs. There are, indeed, many and obvious points of resemblance between the electric organs and the muscles, and, therefore, any interpretation which may be furnished by these organs may be supposed to apply directly, rather than indirectly, to the question under consideration.

What, then, it may be asked, is the process which takes place in the electric organ when it is touched by a foreign body? It is evidently the discharge of electricity previously present. If the fish be touched in a particular manner, a severe shock is the sign of this discharge; but the discharge is not less real when the shock is not felt in this manner. The discharge will indeed take place when the animal is touched by a piece of glass or other non-conductor; or it will take place when the animal is not touched at all, as under the influence of strychnia. This is evident, as well from the continuance of the convulsive movements which accompany every discharge, and particularly from the singular retraction of the eyeballs, as from the exhausted state in which the animal is left after the experiment. In a word, it is not necessary to the discharge that the electricity discharged should extend *beyond* the animal discharging. If fit channels have been provided, the current may extend beyond the animal, and in that case the discharge, with its attendent shock, may be felt accordingly; but if these channels have not been provided the discharge will take place within the animal itself.

And if this be so, the necessary inference is that the electricity of a muscle *may* be discharged indifferently by a conductor or by a non-conductor, for all that is necessary is to suppose that the discharge does not extend beyond the muscle when the non-conductor is used.

Another difficulty is to be found in the fact that muscle contracts with very different degrees of force when it is touched lightly and when it is tapped briskly. When tapped briskly a strong contraction is the result; when touched lightly there may be no contraction at all. In a word, the degree of contraction would seem to be proportionate to the stimulation of the touching or tapping body. It would seem, also, as if these phenomena could not easily be explained on the supposition that some agent like electricity had been discharged, for, according to this view, it may be said that the discharge ought to be equally complete, and the consequent contraction equally marked, when the muscle was touched in the lightest way possible, in that any touch must be sufficient to bring about this discharge. This may be said, but at the same time it is very possible that the tension of the electricity in the muscular fibres may be so low, and the insulation of these fibres so complete, as to require very perfect contact—something more than a light touch—before any discharge can be produced; and it is also possible that the effect of the firmer tap may be to bring more fibres within what may be called discharging distance, and in that way the more marked contraction may be the natural sign of the increased range of the discharge. At any rate, it is very plain that more fibres are made to contract by a sharp tap than by a light touch; for ocular demonstration of this may be had at any time by experimenting upon the surface of any muscle.

A third difficulty may also be disposed of by a little care and consideration. There is no doubt that a muscle will gradually cease to respond to the touch of a foreign body, and that the contractions will not recommence until after an interval of rest; but it does not follow from this fact that there is in the muscle a property of contractility which is exhausted by exercise and recruited by rest. At any rate it is quite as easy to explain the phenomenon upon the hypothesis under consideration. It is easy to suppose that a recently separated muscle will be more quickly charged with electricity than the muscle which has been removed from the body for a longer time, seeing that the molecular changes (respiratory, nutritive, and other), in which the electricity originates or consists, must be more active at first than they are afterwards; and, if so, then it follows that the recently separated muscle will be able to afford a greater number of those *discharges* of which (upon the provisional hypothesis at present under consideration) contraction is the sign. It follows, also, that an interval of time must be necessary to the production of the *charges*—an interval which for many obvious reasons must become continually longer and longer from the time when the muscle is removed from the body to the time when the molecular changes of the muscle come to an end; and hence the result will be precisely as if a vital power of contraction had been fatigued and required to be recruited by rest.

— Nor is the ordinary history of muscular contraction as seen in the vesiculæ seminales, or bladder, or bowel, or uterus, at variance with this mode of interpretation.

If there is one instance in which, more obviously than in any other, mechanical irritation would seem to have acted upon the muscles in the sense of a stimulus, it is in the contractions which take place in the vesiculæ seminales and elsewhere during the sexual orgasm, but even here a very different conclusion may be necessary. In one point of view, indeed, it is even probable that the irritation may have acted by diminishing, and not by increasing, the stimulus derived from the nerves. For what is the case with respect to sensation but this—that each sensation involves a corresponding expenditure of nervous influence and nervous substance? A given amount of nervous influence or nervous substance, so to speak, is used up in each sensation, and after a longer or shorter time the nerve is exhausted and enervated. And so also with the nerve-current. It is not, as might be expected, that this current is intensified at the instant of a sensation. It is a contrary change, for Dr. du Bois-Reymond has found that the current falls whenever the nerve is subjected to a treatment which would give rise to sensation if it remained in connexion with the brain. Thus, the current of the sciatic nerve of a frog is found to fall when the foot is dipped into hot water. Now in the case under consideration, it is not at all difficult to realise this idea and believe that sensation involves a corresponding expenditure of nervous influence, or nerve-current, or nerve-substance; for if there is any case in which exhaustion is the price which has to be paid for sensation, it is this. And if this is the case with respect to sensation, what is it with respect to motion? Is it to be supposed that the irritation which has acted in this manner upon the sensory nerves has acted similarly upon the motor nerves, and that contraction is set up in the vesiculæ seminales, and in other parts of the muscular system, because these motor nerves do not supply the usual amount of nervous influence to the muscles. At any rate, such a supposition cannot be regarded as improbable. On the contrary, there is so intimate a connexion between all parts of the nervous system, and particularly between the sensory and motor nerves belonging to the same part of this system, that it is scarcely possible to suppose that any change of state can be strictly limited to any one part. In pain or pleasure, without any figure, there is indeed no part of the nervous system which does not sympathize with every part, and hence (reasoning from the state of things which is evidently present in the sensory nerves) it is not at all improbable that the explanation of the muscular contractions occurring during the sexual orgasm may be altogether in accordance with the premises.

A similar mode of explanation may also be applied to the contractions by which the bladder or bowel is emptied, for the irritation of the accumulating urine or fæces may be supposed to have brought about the requisite state of enervation in the nerves concerned. At any rate, the uncomfortable feeling of fulness which precedes the contraction may be appealed to as an argument in favour of the idea that the energy of the different afferent nerves is being used up by being converted into sensation.

And, certainly, the doctrine of stimulation is not wanted to explain the parturient contractions of the uterus. At the time of labour this organ returns from the state of progressive expansion in which it had been during the period of pregnancy; and as *one* cause of the previous state of expansion would seem to be found in the increasing vital activity of the fœtus, so now *one* cause of the return from this state would seem to be found in the failure of this activity—a failure brought about, first in the mother, and afterwards in the fœtus, in consequence of the growth of the fœtus having then passed the limit beyond which it cannot pass without trenching upon the supplies necessary for the proper nourishment of the mother. It would seem, also, that this return of the uterus from the expanded state, or, in other words, this contraction of the uterine walls, must compress the vessels going to the placenta,— that the vital activity of the fœtus must suffer a corresponding depression from this interference with the sufficiency of the placental respiration—and that this depression must again lead to contraction in the uterus—for if this organ contracted in the first instance in consequence of a depression of this kind, there is no reason why it should not do so again. And, further, it would seem that this second contraction must lead to a third, and the third to a fourth; and that thus, the uterus acting upon the fœtus, and the fœtus reacting upon the uterus, contraction must follow contraction, until the completion of birth. Nor does it follow from this hypothesis that the uterine contraction should be unintermitting, for it is quite possible (this among other reasons) that the blood which is displaced from the uterus during contraction may temporarily "stimulate" the system of the mother to a degree which is inconsistent with an unintermitting continuance of contraction in any of the muscles belonging to the involuntary system. At any rate, it is quite impossible, upon any rational view of parturition, to refer the contraction of the uterus to any "stimulation" on the part of the fœtus, without ignoring the whole of the previous history of pregnancy.

— Such, then, are the considerations which appear to belong more or less intimately to the present section. They are imperfect, no doubt, and by themselves unsatisfactory, but taken in connection with what has been said in the three preceding sections, they serve to show, if they do no more, that many important difficulties must be done away with before we can conclude that muscle is stimulated to contract by any mechanical agent, natural or artificial.

5. *That muscular contraction is not produced by the stimulation of light.*

Regarding the question generally, contraction would seem to be favoured by darkness rather than by light. It is in the darkness, and not in the light, that contraction takes place in the irritable cushions of the untouched sensitive plant; and it does not seem to be far otherwise with the iris, for it is as easy to suppose that the radiating fibres of this organ elongate under the influence of light, and in that way close the pupil, as to suppose that this curtain is closed by sphincter fibres, which have a very doubtful existence. At all events, this explanation is supported by the authority of Bichât; it equally accounts for the phenomena: and it harmonises with the known influence of light upon the cushions of the sensitive plant.

6. *That muscular contraction is not produced by the stimulation of heat or cold.*

Muscle, it is found, will bear considerable variation of temperature without contracting, but if the temperature be higher or lower than a given point, it is immediately thrown into a state of contraction.

Now, there is reason to believe that the " muscular current " is more or less suspended by a temperature which is higher or lower than a given point, and not by intermediate degrees of temperature, and that the presence or absence of contraction in these experiments may be accounted for by the suspension or non-suspension of the "muscular current." Professor Matteucci has shown that the " muscular current " is suspended by a low temperature, and hence, according to the premises, it is intelligible that the muscle may contract under a sufficient degree of cold. On the other hand, I find that the muscular current is weakened to the last degree, or altogether extinguished by the amount of heat which is sufficient to produce contraction in the muscle. In this experiment I placed the gastrocnemius of a frog across the cushions of the galvanometer, and having laid the end of a small straight band of watch-spring upon it, I raised the temperature of the band by applying a spirit-lamp to the other end. It is intelligible, therefore, that muscle should contract under a temperature which is higher or lower than a given point, and that it should not contract under those intermediate degrees of heat which are not sufficient to weaken the "muscular current" to the point which allows of contraction.

And, certainly, it cannot be said that muscular contraction has been produced by any stimulative action of heat upon the motor nerves, for Dr. Eckardt has recently shown[1] that the effect of the heat is to impair the "irritability" of the nerve, and that the contraction which is caused by heat is coincident with the temporary loss of this "irritability." In this experiment, the leg of a frog is prepared so as to have a long portion of its nerve attached to it, and the irritability of the nerve is tested at different degrees of heat by immersing the nerve in water, the temperature of which may be raised by additions of hot water, and by observing the readiness with which the muscles may be made to contract by irritating the nerve with a needle. The experiment is

[1] Op. cit., p. 81.

simple, and the results are unmistakeable. Thus, in water about the natural temperature of the frog—about 70° Fahr.—the irritability of the nerve is not appreciably affected; in water of a higher temperature the irritability is sensibly impaired by every additional quantity of hot water; at 144° Fahr., or thereabouts, the muscles refuse to respond any longer to the action of the needle upon the nerve; in water at a still higher temperature *the muscles contract in obedience to the action of the hot water upon the nerve.* In other words, the muscle is exhibited as contracting under the influence of heat when the degree of heat is sufficient to have destroyed the irritability of the nerve. Or, as Dr. Eckardt expresses it, " das Zustandekommen der Zuckung durch eine momentane Zerstörung der Structur des Nerven bedingt sei."

— In a word, there is little reason for saying that muscular contraction is produced by the stimulation of heat, and there is scarcely any more reason for thinking that the muscles are ever made to contract under the stimulation of cold.

7. *That muscular contraction is not produced by the stimulation of any chemical or analogous agency.*

The recent investigations of Dr. Harley[1] upon the physiological action of strychnia and brucia

[1] 'Lancet,' June 7th and 14th, and July 12th, 1856.

are calculated to shed much light upon the mode in which muscle is affected by chemical and analogous agencies.

These investigations, which are of extreme importance in a therapeutical as well as in a physiological point of view, show very clearly that these poisons do not cause death by exhaustion, or by suffocation arising either from closure of the glottis, or from spasm in the walls of the chest, but "by destroying the powers of the tissues and fluids of the body to absorb oxygen and give off carbonic acid." It is argued that death is not caused by exhaustion, because it cannot be supposed that the system can be fatally exhausted in less than two minutes. It is proved, that death is not caused by closure of the glottis, because the animal dies as speedily when its windpipe has been freely opened before the administration of the poison. It is proved, moreover, that spasm in the walls of the chest is not the cause of death, because artificial respiration can be performed without averting or even deferring the fatal issue. At the same time, the animal seems to "feel a want of oxygen," and that this is one cause of death Dr. Harley shows very plainly by the examination of its blood.

In this examination Dr. Harley uses the fresh blood of the calf. Of this blood he takes two portions, and mixing a small quantity (0·005 grammes) of strychnia with one, he ascertains the amount of oxygen absorbed and carbonic acid given off by examining the composition of air that has been left in contact with each. In each case the blood is thoroughly saturated with oxygen by shaking it with fresh quantities of air; and after this it is corked up in a graduated tube with 100 per cent. of ordinary air, and frequently agitated for the next twenty-four hours. At the end of this time, the air contained in the tubes is analysed by Bunsen's method, and the following is the result arrived at:

	Composition of common Air.	Composition of Air after having been in contact with *simple blood* for 24 hours	Composition of Air after having been in contact with *blood containing strychnine* for 24 hours.
Oxygen . . .	20·96	11·33	17·82
Carbonic Acid .	·002	5·96	2·73
Nitrogen . .	79·038	82·71	79·45
	100·000	100·00	100 00.

The air, that is to say, which has been in contact with the blood containing strychnia, has more oxygen and less carbonic acid than the air which had been left in contact with simple blood; and thus it would appear, that less oxygen has been absorbed, and less carbonic acid given off by the blood containing strychnine. When brucine is used instead of strychnine, the only difference in the result is one of degree:

	Composition of common Air.	Composition of Air after having been in contact with *simple blood* for 24 hours.	Composition of Air after having been in contact with *blood containing brucine* for 24 hours.
Oxygen . . .	20·96	6·64	11·63
Carbonic Acid .	·002	3·47	2·34
Nitrogen . .	79·038	89·89	86·03
	100·000	100·00	100·00

As with strychnine, therefore, so with brucine, the air which had been left in contact with the poisoned blood, in that it contains more oxygen and less carbonic acid than the air which had been left in contact with the pure blood, has absorbed less oxygen, and given off less carbonic acid than the pure blood.

Dr. Harley has also shown very conclusively that strychnine has, in addition, a direct power of destroying muscular irritability.

In one of these experiments, in which the hearts of two frogs are cut out and placed, one in distilled water, the other in a solution of acetate of strychnine, the result is, that the heart placed in distilled water goes on pulsating regularly for twenty-four hours, and that the heart which had been placed in the poisoned solution, not only ceases to beat in a few minutes (from one to five according to the strength of the solution), but even passes into a state of rigor mortis before the other heart has lost its irritability.

In the other experiment, the hind legs of a frog are prepared after Galvani's method, and placed, one in a vessel containing distilled water, the other in a vessel containing a strong solution of acetate of strychnine. The muscles and nerves of these limbs are separately tested by galvanism, and the result is, that the muscles of the limb immersed in simple water, are seen to contract freely after the muscles of the limb immersed in the poisoned solution have passed into the state of rigor mortis.

The action of the strychnine upon the muscles, indeed, may be supposed to be in some degree analogous to the action upon the blood, for, as Dr. Harley points out, the destruction of the "irritability of the muscle may be supposed to imply the suspension of that process of absorbing oxygen and giving off carbonic acid—the so-called respiration of the muscle—which is certainly most energetic when the irritability is most marked."

At any rate, these very important facts go to show that the action of strychnia, in producing muscular contraction, is not an action of stimulation, for they show that the poison acts first of all by rendering the blood less apt to appropriate its stimulating element, oxygen, and in the second place by diminishing the irritability of the muscles.

In another place, moreover, Dr. Harley says—

"many other poisons, I doubt not, exert their influence in a similar manner; for I have found that hydrocyanic acid, chloroform, nicotine, alcohol, ether, morphine, and several other narcotics, have the same power of destroying the property possessed by the organic constituents of the blood of absorbing oxygen and exhaling carbonic acid."

— An inference as to what really takes place in muscle under the influence of chemical or analogous agencies may also be drawn from Dr. Eckardt's recent experiments upon the "irritability" of the nerves connected with muscle. Experimenting with an acid, for example, it was found that the "irritability" of the nerve was damaged by the application of the acid, and that the muscle was not made to contract *by the acid* unless the concentration of the acid was such as to destroy the "irritability" of the nerve. The experiment, in fact, is the precise counterpart of the one related in the preceding section, the only difference being that an acid of continually increasing strength was employed in this case, and heat of continually increasing intensity in that case. It was the same also in the experiments with other agents. The agents themselves were found to act very differently—some by attracting water from the nerve, some by altering the normal albuminous constituents of the nerve, and some in a more recondite manner—but all agreed in this that they acted by destroying the "irritability" of the nerve, and that they did not cause contraction until they had destroyed this property. The experiments, indeed, appear to show that these agents produce contraction by suspending, and not by exciting, the "irritability."

Nor is any evidence of a contrary character to be met with elsewhere. There is little or no "irritability" in the muscles of animals which have been killed by immersion in carbonic acid, carbonic oxide, hydrogen, sulphurous acid or chlorine—and as little in muscles to which narcotic substances have been applied. The "irritability," moreover, is completely destroyed by the application of concentrated acids or alkalies. On the other hand, the muscles retain their "irritability" for a long time in atmospheric air or oxygen. And this is as might be expected. It has been said, for example, that a muscle *may* contract under the touch of a foreign body, not because it was stimulated to do so, but because the electricity of the muscle was discharged at the time; and that the muscle might cease to contract under these circumstances when the *charge* of electricity necessary to the discharge had ceased to be produced. Hence, loss of "irritability," according to this view, is nothing more than the want of the requisite charge of electricity in the muscle —a view, it may be remarked in passing, which is quite consistent with the supposition that sufficient electricity may still be present in the muscle to counteract the rigidity of death. Now it is quite intelligible that oxygen should be necessary to the development of the full electrical charge of muscle, and hence there is no difficulty in understanding that the muscles should retain their "irritability" for a longer time in atmospheric air or oxygen than in carbonic acid, carbonic oxide, hydrogen, sulphurous acid, or chlorine. It is also intelligible that oxidization should not be the sole source of electrization. The mere contact of dissimilar metals, as zinc and silver in a vacuum or in hydrogen, for example, will give rise to a current. And, therefore, it is possible that there may be such dissimilarities in muscle as may react for a time and give rise to an electrical charge, of feeble tension perhaps, and such as may not be discharged by the touch of a foreign body under ordinary circumstances, but still sufficient to counteract the state of contraction so long as it continues. It is also possible that these dissimilarities may cease after a time—from coagulation of fluids, from desiccation of solids, or from some other cause—and, so ceasing, that contraction may supervene. And, finally, it is possible that a muscle may immediately and effectually lose its power of contracting under the action of strong acids or alkalies, for the physical integrity of the fibre is necessary to contraction upon any hypothesis.

— In a word, it is not necessary to have recourse to the doctrine of stimulation to account for the facts which present themselves for consideration under this section, and there is much reason for believing that muscular contraction is not produced by the stimulation of any chemical or analogous agency.

— Reviewing the whole evidence, then, there appears to be no reason why *rigor mortis* may not be taken as the type of muscular contraction in general. For what is the case with respect to this form of muscular contraction? The case is simply this. As long as there is any trace of that action of which the " muscular current" is a sign, so long is there no *rigor mortis*. As long as there is any trace of that action of which the " nerve current" is a sign, so long is there no *rigor mortis.* If this action dies out speedily, as in persons in whom the vitality of the frame has been exhausted by long life, or by chronic disease, such as consumption, the muscles become speedily rigid; if this action dies out slowly, as in persons who have been cut down suddenly in the full glow of life, the muscles are equally slow in becoming rigid. Once contracted, moreover, the muscles remain contracted until they break up in the ruin of final decay,—an event which happens most speedily in the case where the muscle retains its physical integrity least perfectly. And this is precisely as it should be according to the premises, for according to the premises all that is necessary to the commencement of *rigor mortis* is the cessation of that action of which electricity is a sign, and all that is necessary to its continuance is the absence of this action and the physical integrity of the muscular fibre. In a word, it is possible to explain those unexplained and seemingly contradictory facts which constitute the distinctive features of that contraction into which the muscles pass after death; and hence *rigor mortis* may be accepted, not only as a type of muscular contraction in general, but as an *experimentum crucis* in favour of the proposition —that *muscular contraction is not produced by the stimulation of any contractile power belonging to muscle.*

II. The Second Proposition.

THAT MUSCULAR ELONGATION IS PRODUCED BY THE SIMPLE PHYSICAL ACTION OF CERTAIN AGENTS, ELECTRICITY AND OTHERS, AND THAT MUSCULAR CONTRACTION IS THE SIMPLE PHYSICAL CONSEQUENCE OF THE CESSATION OF THIS ACTION.

In seeking to establish the first proposition we are led, not only to believe that muscular contraction is not produced by the stimulation of any property of contractility belonging to muscle, but we are prepared to go a step further, and accept as probable the proposition which stands at the head of this section. For what is that view of muscular action which arises out of the previous consideration? It is that muscle and the parts more immediately related to muscle are acted upon by certain agents, electricity and others, and that the action is one which antagonizes contraction. It is a view, indeed, in which muscular contraction may be said to change from an active to a passive, from a vital to a physical phenomenon,—for there is nothing which does not seem to be capable of being reducible to a physical explanation. At the same time there are sundry difficulties of a very weighty character, which must be removed before such a view can be accepted.

A grave difficulty arises at the very outset in the fact that a muscle contracts without undergoing any change in volume. In contracting, that is to say, the muscle gains in breadth what it loses in length, and the phenomenon is so peculiar as to seem beyond the scope of any physical explanation.

There are, however, certain changes of a purely physical nature which would seem to approximate in their character to these changes in muscle, and it will be well to consider these. Such, apparently, are the changes which many crystalline bodies undergo under the influence of heat. Under this influence non-crystalline bodies dilate in every direction, becoming both longer and broader in so doing, and this is the case likewise with those crystalline bodies which are singly refractive and of equal axes; but *crystalline bodies (or at least some of them) which are doubly refractive and of unequal axes dilate only in particular directions.* If, for example, a primitive rhomb of calc-spar be heated, it *expands* in the direction of its shortest axis, and *contracts* in the direction perpendicular to the axis. At the same time the rhomb tends to become a cube by a change in its angles in which the obtuse angles become more acute and the acute angles more obtuse. Heated from 32° Fahr. to 212°, according to Mitscherlich and Dulong, the *expansion* of the shorter axis of this crystal of calc-spar is 0·00286, and the *contraction* in the directions perpendicular to this axis

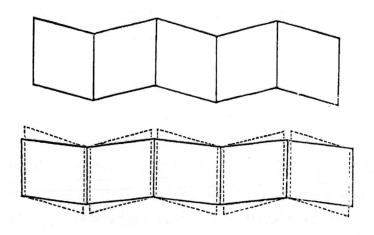

0·00056, so that the relative expansion of the shorter axis is 0·00342 (0·00286 + 0·00056). These changes, which are very curious, may be roughly illustrated by two diagrams, in one of which a series of unexpanded rhombs is arranged longitudinally, and in the other a similar series of rhombs as altered by heat, only with the degree of alteration exaggerated for the sake of distinctness.

— But there is a more direct illustration of the changes in muscular fibre than that which may be found in the changes of calc-spar crystals under the influence of heat, and this is to be found in the changes of a bar of iron under the influence of magnetism. Under the influence of heat the series of crystals increases in length and loses in breadth, and there is little change of volume, but there is some change of volume, and, therefore, the illustration of the changes of muscular fibre is not perfect; but in the bar of iron the illustration is exact, for under the influence of magnetism there is increase of length and loss of breadth, without any alteration of volume. It is to Mr. Joule, of Manchester, that we are mainly indebted for the knowledge of this remarkable fact.[1]

Mr. Joule's experiments are very numerous and exact. The bar of iron was magnetized by placing

[1] 'The Philosophical Magazine,' February and April, 1857.

it in the axis of a coil of insulated copper wire, and by then passing a current of electricity through the coil. One end of the bar was fixed; the other end was attached to a system of levers by which any change in length was multiplied 3000 times. In one experiment a bar of rectangular iron wire, two feet long, one fourth of an inch broad, and one eighth of an inch thick, was placed in a coil of twenty-two inches in length and one third of an inch in diameter, and the result of the experiment was, that when the coil was traversed by the current of a battery capable of magnetizing the bar to saturation, or nearly so, the index of the multiplying apparatus sprang from its position and vibrated about a point one tenth of an inch in advance—a distance which gave $\frac{1}{30000}$th of an inch as the actual elongation of the bar. After a short interval the index ceased to vibrate, and began to advance very gradually in consequence of the expansion of the bar under the heat radiating from the coil; and this it did until the circuit was broken, when it immediately began to vibrate about a point exactly one tenth of an inch lower than that to which it had attained. On examining the end of the bar with a microscope the elongation or shortening of the bar was seen to take place with extreme suddenness. In other experiments it was found that the elongation was in the duplicate ratio of the magnetic intensity of the bar, and (for the same intensity of magnetism) that it was in direct proportion to the softness of the metal, being greatest in well-annealed iron and least in hardened steel.

In order to show that the bar of iron underwent no change of volume under these circumstances, Mr. Joule placed a bar of annealed iron, one yard long and half an inch square, in a glass tube, forty inches long and an inch and a half in diameter, around which an insulated conductor, consisting of ten copper wires, each 110 yards long and one twentieth of an inch in diameter, had been previously coiled. One extremity of this tube was sealed hermetically; the other was fitted with a stopper, which had been perforated so as to allow the insertion of a graduated capillary tube. The bulk of the iron bar was 4,500,000 times the capacity of each division of the graduated capillary tube. In performing an experiment, the tube was filled with water, the stopper adjusted, the capillary tube inserted so as to force the water to a convenient height within it, and the coil connected with a Daniell's battery of five or six cells—an apparatus of sufficient power to magnetize the iron bar to the full—and the invariable result was that no perceptible change of level was produced either on making or on breaking contact with the battery, and that equally whether the water was stationary in the capillary tube, or whether it was rising or falling from any change of temperature in the bar. The experiment, indeed, afforded most conclusive proof that the bar underwent no change of *bulk* on being magnetized, for if the elongation of the bar under these circumstances had not been accompanied by a corresponding decrease in breadth, the water would have been forced through twenty divisions of the capillary tube whenever the circuit of the battery was completed.

By other experiments Mr. Joule found that these results were greatly modified under certain circumstances. He found, indeed, that under a certain degree of *tension*, an iron wire, instead of becoming longer, actually became shorter, when magnetized; but under ordinary circumstances the results were as have been stated.

— The changes which take place in a bar of iron under the influence of magnetism are paralleled, therefore, by the changes which take place in muscular fibre, for while the fibre increases in length, and loses in breadth, under the influence of electricity and its associate agencies, and loses in length and gains in breadth when this influence is withdrawn, so likewise does the bar of iron increase in length and lose in breadth under the influence of electricity, and lose in length and gain in breadth when this influence is withdrawn. And not only is this parallelism preserved in the changes of shape and in the agencies concerned, but it is preserved in that point which is so characteristic of muscle, namely, the *suddenness* with which the contracted and elongated states may alternate upon each other,—for in Mr. Joule's experiments the bar was seen and heard and felt to *jump* into the longer form, and then to jump back again into the shorter form, as the electricity was communicated to or withdrawn from the coil.

— There are, however, certain facts which, at first sight, do not appear to be altogether consistent with this physical mode of regarding the phenomena of muscular contraction. How, for instance, can we explain that diminished degree of shortening which is noticed when a muscle contracts after death, except upon the supposition that the contractile power is a vital endowment? How is that loss of contractile power which is consequent upon death to be otherwise accounted for? How is it that the muscle loses in power as it contracts upon itself? How is it that the muscle wastes in proportion to the number of its contractions, without supposing that the contraction is the sign of functional activity in the muscle?

There is no doubt that a muscle contracts most perfectly during life, but this does not prove that the diminished degree of contraction which is noticed after death is owing to the loss of some vital power of contraction. On the contrary, there is no good reason why this diminished degree of shortening after death may not be the natural result of the peculiar circumstances in which the muscle is then placed. When a muscle contracts during life, the antagonist muscle either relaxes, or opposes no resistance to the contraction. The blood, also, is fluid, and the intra-muscular vessels are easily emptied when pressed upon by the contracting fibres. But after death the spasm is universal, and the contraction of any set of muscles is not favoured by the relaxation of the antagonist set. After death, moreover, the full degree of muscular contraction may be prevented by the coagulated contents of some of the intra-muscular vessels. At the same time it must not be forgotten, that muscle may contract to a very considerable extent after death, and that this is the case in any muscle when the antagonist muscle has been divided.

Nor is the loss of muscular strength after death a necessary proof that the contractile power of muscle is a vital endowment. On the contrary, loss of strength may, or rather must be, the natural consequence of the peculiar circumstances in which the muscle is then placed. In the first place, the fibre may be acted upon by those solvent juices which are present in muscle, and which are more or less analogous in their properties to gastric juice; and, if so, then the fibre may be partially dissolved after death, and to that extent weakened. In the second place, the dead muscle is yielded up to the processes of decomposition, and the affinities of the *muscular* molecules may be weakened by resolution of these molecules into their constituent elements; and hence another reason why the dead muscular fibre may have suffered some loss of strength,—and this, not because the contractile power of muscle is a vital endowment, but simply because this power requires for its full manifestation a physical integrity of the muscular fibre, which no longer exists.

It is true, also, that the muscle contracts with diminished power as it contracts upon itself, but this is no objection to the idea that muscular contraction is a physical phenomenon. On measuring the force with which the muscles of a frog's leg contracted at different degrees of shortening, M. Schwann found that the force decreases as the fibres become shortened; and finding this, and supposing that the force of the contraction should increase after a definite law as the fibre contracts if the contraction were due to any known physical attractive force, he inferred that muscular contraction could not be due to any such force; but he overlooked the fact, that the non-contracting or imperfectly contracting cellular substance of the muscle, and the comparatively inelastic fluids contained in the muscle, may oppose such *resistance* to the contraction of the proper muscular fibres as to mask the pure law of that contraction, and, overlooking this, his inference has not even a shadow of foundation. This experiment may indeed show the *degree of resistance* which is opposed to muscular contraction; but it is altogether worthless as an argument in support of the idea that the law of muscular contraction is essentially different from the law of physical attractive forces,—indeed elastic bodies, in shrinking after elongation, behave in every respect as muscle behaves in this experiment, and here, unquestionably, this shrinking must be a physical process.

And, lastly, it is more than doubtful whether the inference to be drawn from the fact that the waste of a muscle is proportionate to the amount of muscular action is—that muscular contraction is the sign of functional activity in the muscle. It is more than doubtful, indeed, whether this waste can be directly related to the contraction even by a vicious process of reasoning. On the other hand, it is not at all improbable that this waste may have been incurred, not in producing but in counteracting contraction, for it is certain that that electrical state which, according to the premises, is concerned in counteracting contraction, cannot be kept up without a corresponding change,—that is, waste, in the tissues concerned.

— And if these objections may be overruled, then there is no longer any sufficient reason for continuing to believe that a vital property of contractility—whether of irritability or of tonicity—has anything to do with muscular contraction. On the contrary there is every reason for discarding such an idea. For what has been the unvarying drift of the argument? It has led us to regard the elongated rather than the contracted state as the chief peculiarity of muscle, and it has seemed to show that any vital property of muscle, if such there be, must be exercised in counteracting rather than in favouring contraction. It has seemed to show that living muscle is acted upon by certain agents, electricity and others; that this action antagonizes contraction; that the transitory contractions which are said to belong to that form of contractility which is called *irritability* occur in transitory lulls of this action; and that the persistent contraction of *rigor mortis*, which is referred to that form of contractility which is called *tonicity*, is persistent because the action which antagonizes contraction has then died out. The unvarying drift of the argument, indeed, has seemed to show that a property like contractility would hinder rather than help. In a word, the only conclusion to which we have been able to arrive is one which excludes altogether from the phenomena of muscular action the idea of a vital property of contractility and the doctrine of stimulation which is founded upon it,—for this doctrine implies the existence of this property.

It is, no doubt, a difficult matter to abandon an idea which has been so long fixed in the mind as the idea that a vital property of contractility belongs to muscle, and that that property is stimulated into action when the muscle contracts. It is difficult to believe that the final purpose of a muscle—its contraction, and particularly that form of contraction which is obedient to the mandates of the will, instead of being brought about by the infusion of more life into the muscle, should be brought about by a change which is realised to its fullest extent in *rigor mortis*. At the same time the difficulty, such as it is, diminishes when it is steadily looked in the face. So far as the will is concerned, it does not follow that this principle should be ever other than an active vital power; and the only change required is to suppose that the will should bring about muscular contraction, not by imparting something to the muscle, but by suspending something which had previously antagonized contraction. The idea changes with reference to the muscle, but not with reference to the will, for in either case the will must *act*. And as to the rest, it is surely more easy to suppose that the will acts through the instrumentality of a force which belongs to muscle as a physical structure than it is to suppose that it can only act through the instrumentality of a superadded property of contractility, and a special apparatus for stimulation.

— Instead of being vital and peculiar, therefore, muscular elongation would not seem to differ essentially from that elongation which takes place in a bar of iron under the action of the electric current; instead of being vital and peculiar, muscular contraction would not seem to differ essentially from the contraction which takes place in the same bar when the action of the electric current is withdrawn; and, if so, then there is no reason why we may not accept the second proposition, which is—*that muscular elongation is due to the simple physical action of certain agents, electricity and others, and that muscular contraction is the simple physical consequence of the cessation of this action.*[1]

---

[1] In these remarks the attention has been confined to the movements of muscular tissue, but there is no reason why the movements of all irritable tissues, the simplest as well as the most complex, should not be obedient to the same law. There is no reason, for example, why such movements as are seen in

III. The Third Proposition.

That the special muscular movements which are concerned in carrying on the circulation—the rhythm of the heart and those movements of the vessels which are independent of the heart—are susceptible of a physical explanation when they are interpreted upon the previous view of muscular action.

1. It is difficult to read the riddle of the heart's action, but the task is not a little simplified when Protozoa, like the Amæba, or in a common colourless corpuscle of the blood, should not be produced in the same manner as the movements of the muscles in the hand of man. Dr. du Bois-Reymond has shown that all organized structures, so far as they have been examined, are the seat of electrical action, and therefore there is no difficulty in assuming that the coats of the Amæba or of the colourless corpuscle of the blood are under the influence of electrical action, or rather are under the influence of a force which in one of its manifestations is called electricity, that elongation of certain parts may be the effect of this action, and that contraction may follow when this action is suspended. At any rate, it is as easy to make this assumption as to suppose that elongation is produced by a process of which we know nothing, and that contraction is brought about by the aid of a property of contractility through the aid of a process of stimulation of which we know less than nothing. A fact, moreover, has just been brought to light by Dr. Macdonnell, of Dublin, which seems to show that there is actually a discharge of electricity when the tentacles of an Actinia are touched by a foreign body, and in this

the previous view of muscular motion is made to serve as a key.

Upon any existing theory of muscular action it is more than difficult to understand why the *ventricles* remain distended with blood during the full half of the rhythmic period, if the *ventricular systole* is in anywise called into existence by the stimulation of the blood; but this fact is not altogether unintelligible if, on the contrary, it be supposed (as must be supposed upon the previous view of muscular action) that the office of the blood will rather be to antagonise the systole and induce the diastole. Indeed upon this view the difficulty appears to be at an end, for according to it the

---

way we are brought to a point from which we can, as it were, look directly into those changes of form which are exhibited in the processes put out from the Amæba, or colourless corpuscle of the blood. Indeed, every Actinia passes through a rudimentary condition which differs in no essential particular from that in which the protozoon, or corpuscle is permanently fixed. The fact which has been brought to light is this—that the muscles of a frog's limb, prepared in the manner which is called the rheoscopic limb, are thrown into a state of contraction when the end of the nerve is brought into contact with one of the tentacles of the Actinia, or even when a metallic conductor is interposed in a particular manner between the tentacle and the nerve. The fact is one, indeed, which seems to show that the tentacles were charged with electrical force, and that a discharge of this force took place when they were touched, for, after what has been said elsewhere, it may be assumed that such a discharge is indicated by the contractions in the frog's limb.

ventricles are thrown into the state of diastole by the stimulation of the blood which has been injected into the coronary system of vessels, and they remain in this state until this blood has given up its arterial properties and so ceased to be stimulating. And certain it is that the different action of the ventricles in anæmia and plethora is calculated to strengthen this idea. Thus: in plethora the pulse (which is the direct test of the action of the ventricles) is full and slow; in anæmia it is small and quick. In the one case, that is to say, the ventricle fills to distension with rich blood and the systole is deferred—in the other case, the ventricle takes in a small quantity of poor unstimulating blood, and the systole follows with scarcely any delay. The facts, indeed, are the very opposites of what they would be found to be if the blood stimulated the ventricle to contract, for in that case the pulse must be small and quick in plethora, and full and slow in anæmia. But if, on the other hand, the blood provokes the ventricle to the diastole by causing elongation in the muscular fibres composing this chamber, then it is intelligible that the ventricle should dilate more fully and the dilatation continue for a longer time, when the blood is rich and warm as in plethora, than when it is poor and watery, as in anæmia.

It may also be presumed that the ventricle is

not stimulated to contract by "nervous influence." At any rate, this would appear to be the inference which may be drawn from the effects of fear upon the pulse. Thus: when the nervous influence is more or less depressed from this cause the heart beats quickly and yet little blood is propelled into the vessels. The beats are perhaps doubled, and yet the skin is cold and pale. Now, under ordinary circumstances, the double number of beats would propel a double quantity of blood into the vessels, and the skin would be hot and red instead of cold and pale; and hence the inference arising out of this anomalous state of the rapid pulse and cold skin attending upon fear is that the ventricular diastole is less complete, and that on that account, a less amount of blood is pumped out of the heart than usual. In other words, the ventricle would seem to have contracted coincidentally with a withdrawal of nervous influence, for some of this influence may be supposed to be withdrawn from the system during fear.

On realising the phenomena of the heart's action more distinctly it becomes even still more improbable that the systole of the venticle is caused by any kind of stimulation, and of the blood more particularly. For what are the facts? At the systole the blood rushes through the coronary arteries into the coats of the heart, and the diastole of the ventricles is attendant upon this rush. And after the blood has remained in these coats until it may be supposed to have lost some of it arterial properties, then the systole returns. These are the simple facts; and thus if stimulation has to do with the phenomena at all it is with the diastole and not with the systole.

It appears, indeed, as if the *ventricular diastole* were due, partly to the force with which the blood is injected into the coronary arteries at the ventricular systole, and partly to the elongating, electro-motive effects of the arterial blood upon the cardiac fibres. It appears, also, as if the diastole of the ventricles were made to continue as long as the blood retained its arterial properties, and that the systole returned when the oxygen was exhausted and the arterial converted into venous blood. And thus, it appears as if the rhythm of the ventricles had a *part* of its explanation, for according to this view, so long as the proper blood continues to be supplied, and so long as the ventricle continues to be capable of responding to it, so long must the systole give rise to the diastole, and the diastole be followed by the systole.

A little further examination will also serve to show that the *systole of the auricles* must be contemporaneous with the *diastole of the ventricle,* for this *systole of the auricles*, there is reason to believe, is, in great measure, the mere *falling in* of the auricular walls upon the sudden withdrawal of blood from the auricles by the diastole of the ventricles. There is reason for this opinion in the absence of valves at the mouths of the veins opening into the auricles, and the reason is obvious. For if the auricles had to contract primarily like the ventricles, is it not fair to assume that there would have been valves to prevent the reflux of the blood from the auricles into the great veins? And if so, then there is no difficulty in accounting for the rhythm of the auricles, for the *auricular diastole*, which is virtually coincident with the ventricular diastole, will be partly due to the same cause as the ventricular diastole, namely, the rush of blood into the coronary system of arteries, and partly to the onward current of blood which is continually setting in from the veins; and the *auricular systole* will be *mainly* due to the collapse of the auricular walls upon the sudden passage of blood into the ventricles at the ventricular diastole.

— But how, it may be asked, will this explanation accord with the known fact that the heart will go on beating after it is removed from the body, and that a mere fragment of the heart will often continue to beat for some time under the same circumstances?

It is a well known fact that the heart of many animals will beat for some time after removal from the body, and that a fragment even may continue to beat regularly under these circumstances; but it is not every fragment that has this power. If, for example, as Mr. Paget reminds us in the admirable and philosophical Croonian Lecture[1] recently delivered before the Royal Society, the cut-out heart of a tortoise be divided into two pieces, the one comprising the auricles and the base of the ventricle, the other comprising the rest of the ventricles, the former piece will go on acting rhythmically, but not the latter piece. Not that the latter piece has lost its capacity for contraction, for it contracts vigorously when touched with any foreign body, but when touched in this manner it contracts once and no more, like any ordinary muscle. Or, if the ventricle of a frog's heart be separated, and all traces of the auricles removed, so that its cavity is perfectly simple; and if this ventricle, so separated, be set upright upon a board with some blood in its cavity and around it, it will be found to pulsate less and less frequently as pieces are snipped away from its upper border; and after a zone of a certain depth (nearly one third of the length of the ventricle) has been snipped away,

---

[1] 'On the Cause of the Rhythmic Motion of the Heart,' Proc. of R. Society, May 28th, 1857.

it will cease to pulsate altogether. It appears, indeed, as if the rhythmically acting heart may be reduced to the region which intervenes between the auricle and the ventricle, and that every part of this region had this power, for every fragment, be it ever so small, will beat regularly for some time. Again: if, in a tortoise or frog, a ligature be tied tightly around the great veins at their line of insertion into the auricle, the rhythmic action of the heart ceases either immediately or presently, and then returns in the ventricles alone: but, if the veins be tied at some distance from the auricles, the rhythm continues. In the experiment, also, where the ligature embraces the veins at their line of insertion into the auricles, it is found that there is a rhythmic motion in the veins behind the ligature, but not the same motion as that which is exhibited in the ventricles.

It is evident, then, as Mr. Paget argues, that the origin of the rhythmic motion of the heart is not in the muscular structure alone, and the inference is that certain nerves and nerve-centres are concerned in it, for the dissections of Bidder and Rosenberger have shown that the region between the auricles and ventricles, and the neighbourhood of the mouths of the great veins are especially rich in nerves. And that nerves are concerned in it would also appear in the fact that the rhythmic actions of respiration (as many experiments show) are connected, not only with the muscular apparatus, but also with the system of nerves whose centre is the medulla oblongata.

Such, then, being the anatomical conditions of the rhythm when the heart is removed from the body, or when a mere fragment is concerned, the question returns which was asked before,—how is this rhythm to be explained?

Now, according to Mr. Paget, this rhythm is due to "time-regulated discharges of nerve force in certain of the ganglia in and near the substance of the heart, by which discharges the muscular walls are excited to contraction," and these time-regulated discharges are themselves due to the *nutrition* of the ganglia and contractile tissues being rhythmic, that is, to these ganglia and contractile tissues "being, in certain periods, by nutritive changes of composition, raised, with regulated progress, to a state of instability of composition, in their decline from which they discharge nerve-force, or change their shape in contracting." Now it is more than probable that certain periodical changes in *nutrition* are concerned in producing the action of the heart, and that, without these, this action must soon come to an end; but at the same time we incline to think that changes which must be referred to *respiration* rather than to nutrition, are those which are

directly concerned in the production of the rhythm.
Indeed, there appears to be no manner of reason
why the same principles of explanation which have
been applied to the ordinary movement of the heart
should not be applicable also to the movement of
the heart or a fragment of the heart out of the
body. In the explanation already given, the idea
was that the oxygen of the arterial blood, injected by the systole of the left ventricle, and
acting upon the muscular and nervous elements
of the coats of the heart, produced the diastole
by rousing (among other things) the muscular
and nerve currents, or, in other words, by
rousing the polar condition of the muscular and
nervous fibres; and that the systole followed the
diastole, in consequence of the failure of these currents, when the arterial blood had parted with its
oxygen, and so ceased to be sufficiently stimulating. And if, under ordinary circumstances, the
blood acts in this manner, then there appears to
be no great difficulty in understanding how it is that
the heart, or a portion of the heart, may go on
pulsating after removal from the body. For why
should oxygen dissolved in the blood act differently from oxygen diffused in the air? Why, for
instance, should not the air, which bathes the surface and permeates every interstice, provoke a
diastolic state in the separate heart or a fragment

of the same, by rousing that polar condition which in the nerves and muscles is designated under the name of the nerve and muscular currents? Why may not the systolic state supervene upon this diastolic state when the polar condition fails, in consequence, as it were, of the arterial air having become converted into venous air? And why, again, should not the diastole return after every systole, so long, that is, as the muscle is capable of responding to the action of the oxygen, for it may well be supposed that the commotion of the systole will displace the venous air and bring the muscular and nervous tissues into relation with fresh quantities of arterial air? Assuredly there is no evident reason to the contrary, and there is one reason why this view should be received, and this is to be found in the fact that the rhythm is rendered more rapid, and even revived for some time after its actual cessation, by placing the heart in oxygen instead of atmospheric air, and that it is brought to a stop by placing the heart in a vacuum or by immersing it in hydrogen or nitrogen or carbonic acid.

It may be assumed, also, that the same view is no less applicable to the explanation of other kinds of rhythmic motion, for it is easy to perceive that these different forms may depend, on the one hand, on differences of structure—differences in the kind of irritable fibre or substance, in the presence or absence of nerves, in the number of blood-vessels, or in the amount of exposed surface,—and, on the other hand, upon the different rates and degrees of oxidization which are consequent upon these differences of structure.

— According to this view, therefore, there need be no difficulty in explaining the rhythm of the heart in accordance with the previous view of muscular action, and the fact that the heart, or a portion of the heart, will go on pulsating for some time after removal from the body, instead of being an objection to this view, may even be an additional argument in its favour.

2. Nor is it easy to understand how it is that the circulation is carried on, if the vessels contract under the influence of certain stimuli acting upon them. If the blood stimulates the vessels to contract, there seems to be only one conclusion, and this is, that the contraction must impede the entrance of blood into the vessels; and so likewise with every other stimulus. But if the blood antagonizes contraction, this difficulty is at an end, and a key may be obtained to the interpretation of those mysterious movements of the blood which are independent of the action of the heart. And this view, which is deducible from the premises, is also warranted by the facts which have still to be mentioned. When the blood is rich and stimulating, as in plethora,

the vessels are red and full; when the blood is poor and watery, as in anæmia, the vessels are shrunk and empty. When the "nervous energy" is exuberant, as in joyous excitement, the skin is flushed; when the nervous energy is depressed, as during fear, the skin is pale. When the hand is held to the fire it flushes with blood; when exposed to cold it becomes blanched and bloodless. The facts, indeed, are utterly inconsistent with the idea that the muscular coats of the vessels are stimulated to contract by blood, or nervous influence, or heat,— and these facts are only examples of many others which might be adduced; but they are not inconsistent with the idea that the contracted state of the vessels is antagonized by the action of these so-called "stimuli."

Now, it follows from the premises that elongation of the vascular muscular fibres and consequent expansion of the vessel itself, may result from the admission of arterial blood into a vessel, and that in this way the admission of blood into a vessel may lead to the admission of more blood, until the vascular fibres have elongated to the full extent required by the amount of oxygen contained in the blood; and, if so, then it may be supposed that the blood will have the power of making for itself a way into and through the vessels—a power which will be in direct proportion to its arterial properties.

And certainly this view is in accordance with the facts which have been mentioned as well as with the facts which remain to be noticed. Indeed, it will afford the only explanation of such purely vascular movements as are exemplified in "*determination of blood*" and in those *ever-shifting-to-and-fro-movements* which are seen in the vascular area of animals before the formation of a heart, or in the laticiferous vessels of plants.

When the hand is held to the fire the heat will produce expansion of the vessels, partly by rousing the polar action of the vascular fibres, and partly by its direct expansive influence upon the areolar and other simple textures; and this expansion will necessitate "*determination of blood*" to the part. It is supposable, also, that the additional quantity of blood which is thus received into the expanded vessels will rouse the nerves of the part into fuller action, and that this fuller action, reacting upon the nervous centres, will lead to further expansion of the vessels, and further admission of blood into them, by augmenting, so to speak, the polar tension of the vascular coats. And hence, reasoning in this manner, "determination of blood" to the part is the necessary consequence of holding the hand to the fire.

Nor does the same principle of interpretation fail when applied to the *ever-shifting-to-and-fro move-*

ments of the "vascular area" of animals before the formation of the heart, or of the laticiferous vessels of plants. Now these fugitive centres of fluctuating movement occur in a web of vessels of unequal sizes; and it is this fact which appears to be concerned in the explanation of the difficulty. Assuming, indeed, that the reaction between the vessels and their contents will be proportionate to the extent of the coats and the quantity of the contents, and that for this reason the larger vessels will experience a greater degree of expansion than the smaller,—it follows that the largest vessels will tend to become still larger, and that they will go on expanding and filling until a limit is reached in which the elongating fibres of the vessels are elongated to the full extent of which they are physically capable under the "stimulus" supplied; and that after this the vessels next in size, because next in size, will expand and fill (partly at the expense of the fluid contained in the vessels which have already filled to their full extent, and partly at the expense of the fluid contained in the emptier vessels) until they can expand and fill no more. It follows, indeed, that the scene of expansion and filling will continually change to the vessels next in size, when the vessels already expanding are full, and that this transference of action will continue as long as the field of action consists of vessels of unequal sizes. As long as the field of action consists of vessels of unequal sizes,—for it is manifest that there could be none of those inequalities of action which, according to the hypothesis, are concerned in the production of these fugitive hearts if the vessels of the web were of the same size in every part.

— In this way, then, it appears to be possible to explain those special and peculiar muscular actions which are concerned in carrying on the circulation—the rhythm of the heart, and those movements of the vessels which are independent of the heart—and as this way is that which naturally arises out of the premises, this very fact may be taken as an additional argument in favour of the correctness of that view of muscular action which is set forth in the two previous sections of this inquiry.

EPILEPSY

AND

OTHER CONVULSIVE AFFECTIONS;

THEIR PATHOLOGY AND TREATMENT.

EPILEPSY,

ETC. ETC.

EPILEPSY is at once the great type of convulsive disorders, and the key to their interpretation. Epilepsy, however, is a name which indicates much less than it did formerly. Thus, it does not indicate the epileptiform convulsion which is connected with certain positive diseases of the brain, with fever, with certain suppressed excretions, with "irritation" in the gums and elsewhere, or with the moribund state; and it is difficult to say what it does indicate, for as our diagnosis gains in exactness, epilepsy changes more and more from a special malady into a mere symptom. At the same time, it is, and, in all probability, it always will be, convenient to take an ideal type of epilepsy and regard it as a special malady, for there are, and ever must be, numberless cases in which, in their earlier stages at least, it will be very difficult, if not impossible, to recognise the disease of which the convulsion is merely a symptom.

Passing from this ideal form of epilepsy to the

consideration of the actual disorders in which muscular contraction is in excess, it is found that these disorders may be conveniently divided into three categories, of which the distinctive signs are—tremor, convulsion, and spasm; but it must not be forgotten that such division is purely arbitrary, and that spasm, convulsion, and tremor, are continually occurring in the same case, and at the same time.

The first category, in which the muscular disturbance takes the form of tremor, is that which includes the tremors of delicate and aged persons, of paralysis agitans, of delirium tremens, the rigors and subsultus of fevers, as well as the tremblings of slow mercurial poisoning.

The second category, in which convulsion is the distinctive feature of the muscular disturbance, may be divided into two sections by the absence or presence of consciousness during the convulsions. Where the consciousness is present the convulsion may be called *simple;* where the consciousness is absent, it is *epileptiform.* Simple convulsion is that which is met with in the state called hysteria, in chorea, and in those strange affections which take an intermediate position between the two, as the dance of St. Vitus and St. John, tarantism, and other affections of the kind. Epileptiform convulsion includes the convulsions connected with certain diseases of the brain,—chronic softening, chronic meningitis, tumour, induration, hypertrophy, atrophy, congestion, apoplexy, inflammation—with fever, with certain suppressed excretions, with "irritation" in the gums and elsewhere, and with the moribund state.

The third category, in which prolonged muscular contraction or spasm is the distinctive state, includes catalepsy, tetanus, cholera, hydrophobia, ergotism, the rigidity of cerebral paralysis, the spasm connected with certain diseases of the spinal cord, and some other spasms of a minor character.

The several chapters, as suggested by the previous considerations, will be—

Chapter I. Of Simple Epilepsy.
Chapter II. Of Tremor.
Chapter III. Of Simple Convulsion.
Chapter IV. Of Epileptiform Convulsion.
Chapter V. Of Spasm.

CHAPTER I.

OF SIMPLE EPILEPSY.

In considering this subject the points successively attended to will be—the general history of the epileptic, the history of the paroxysm, the appearances after death, the pathology (as deduced, first, from a consideration of the phenomena connected with the vascular system, and, secondly, from a consideration of the phenomena connected with the nervous system), and, last of all, the treatment.

1. *The general history of the epileptic.*

An epileptic will often say—never oftener, perhaps, than upon the very eve of a fit—" I am quite well," and others are ready enough to echo what he says; but in every instance there is something wanting which is necessary to warrant this statement.

Where the malady has not made much progress, there may be a cheerful countenance, a sharp digestion, a firm limb, and at the first glance it may not be easy to say what is wanting, but however masked, there are certain signs which are not compatible with true health and strength. In very many instances there is a want of fire in the countenance, and a dilated and sluggish state of the pupil, which point to the brain as lacking in energy; and in keeping with these signs, it is found, on inquiry, that the memory is more or less treacherous, the ideas more or less indefinite, the powers of attention more or less incapable, the imagination more or less dull, the temper more or less irritable, the will more or less feeble, the character more or less undecided. It is no doubt common enough to meet with epileptics who, without any want of candour on their part, will maintain that their minds are free from all infirmity; but if care be taken to examine their history, it will always be found that they and their friends have very different opinions on this subject.

In very many instances there is a marked disposition to tremulousness and cramps; thus, in upwards of seventy cases which fell under the notice of my friend and colleague, Dr. Reynolds,[1] these symptoms occurred at one time or another, and in one form or another, in more than half of the whole number.

In very many instances, again, if not in all, the hands and feet are cool or cold, the pulse is scarcely

---

[1] 'Lancet,' 4th and 11th August, 1855.

ever otherwise than weak and slow, and a feeling of chilliness is almost habitual. Indeed, so far as my own experience goes, the powers of the circulation are always defective, and I do not remember a single instance of a person suffering from simple epilepsy who had the red lips and face, the full pulse and distended veins of plethora, or even a faint semblance of such a state, except, perhaps, for a short time after the fit. For a short time after a convulsion, there may be some degree of reaction in the circulation, but if there be it soon dies out, and the state which follows it is more akin to collapse than plethora. I know, indeed, of cases presenting satisfactory evidences of plethora, in which apoplexy and paralysis were the dangers to be apprehended, and in which epileptiform convulsions were the occasional accompaniments of the apoplectic or paralytic state; but these convulsions, as will be shown eventually, are not to be confounded with those of ordinary epilepsy, without confounding matters, practical as well as theoretical, which ought to be carefully kept apart.

In confirmed cases, these general features are so marked as to be altogether unmistakeable. Not only are the pupils dilated and sluggish, but the under eyelids may have become puffy and coarse. The complexion, moreover, has often acquired a dull tinge—a change which appears to depend in part upon an habitually bloodshot condition of the skin. At any rate, this bloodshot condition is rarely absent, and where it is most marked, as about the forehead and eyelids, it is often accompanied by numerous spots of ecchymosis of about the size of a pin's head. The torpid features are now rarely lighted up with the fire of feeling or thought, the senses are duller than ever, the memory more treacherous, the ideas more confused, the power of attention more distracted, the imagination more drowsy, the temper more uneven, the will more powerless. At this time, also, there is, for the most part, little of that fine susceptibility of feeling which is necessary to enable one to be miserable about anything.

This change for the worse is particularly marked after the fit. Indeed, at this time the senses may be so blunted, and the mind so clouded and confused, that the features of the epileptic may become identical with those of the demented person. Or symptoms of mental aberration may take the place of those which belong to the demented state, and the general features of the epileptic may merge into those of the lunatic. The fits, also, may recur so frequently, that the mind may never have the chance of clearing up in the interval, and in this way the same general features may never cease to be confounded with those of the demented or insane person.

Not unfrequently, also, there is the very gravest degree of mental infirmity from the very first, and instead of ending in dementia, the history of the epileptic may begin in idiotcy. Indeed, epilepsy is so frequent an accompaniment of this saddest of all deplorable conditions, that it can scarcely be said to be an accident.

— The causes of epilepsy, so far as we know, are also in accordance with the foregoing considerations.

A very common cause is hereditary predisposition. In other words, the bodily and mental features which have been described are transmitted, not acquired. And all this is intelligible enough, for it is much more easy to understand that the offspring should be like the parent than unlike the parent.

Epilepsy is very often referred to fright or fear, and this fact is also a collateral argument in favour of the previous considerations: for, in order that fright or fear should operate in this inordinate manner, it is necessary that there should be some undue weakness or want of balance in the system. It is necessary that a man should incline to the feminine type, or that a woman should retain too much of the impressibility of childhood.

Another and very important inducing cause is sexual abuse of one kind or another. All are agreed upon this point, and all are also agreed that this cause is one which produces no ordinary degree of exhaustion.

Over-study is also an occasional, but by no means a frequent, predisposing cause. I have met with several instances where over-study may have helped to bring out a latent predisposition, but I know of no case in which it could be said to be a principal, or even important cause.

Of the causes which bring on the individual attacks I should be disposed to mention undue muscular exercise as one of the most frequent. At any rate I have notes of several cases in which the fits diminished in number, or remained in abeyance altogether, so long as the patient was careful to avoid any fatigue, and where a fit was almost sure to follow any carelessness in this respect.

After muscular fatigue, I would lay most stress upon abstinence. Epileptics, so far as my experience goes, bear abstinence ill, and I have often been surprised at the rapidity with which they become faint, if they are kept waiting beyond the time of their accustomed meal.

And after abstinence I should be disposed to mention sexual imprudence as a cause to which the individual attacks may often be referred.

Nor is a different conclusion to be drawn from the fact, that the fits have a marked tendency to recur at particular periods. They recur, for example, in the night rather than in the day, and they do not recur indifferently at all periods of the month or year. I cannot enter upon this subject here, and all I can say is, that this *periodicity* (as I have endeavoured to show elsewhere)[1] is only one among many of the signs of defective vital power. The plant exhibits plainer and more numerous evidences of periodicity than the animal; and it does this, I argue, because it has less of that innate life which enables man and the higher animals to be partially independent of the sun and other vivifying influences which act upon them from without; and hence it follows (this among other reasons) that the man who exhibits more evidences of periodicity than he ought to do, has been shorn of some of that innate life which is the badge of distinction between him and the plant.

— In a word, the features of the epileptic are always of a cheerless character, and even where they are least marked, they show that the epileptic has no right to say "I am quite well."

2. *The history of the epileptic paroxysm.*

The signs of the approaching paroxysm are very variable. The patient himself will generally say, and say truly, that the fit takes him by surprise, and certainly the signs of danger are not those

---

[1] First edition of this work, chap. iii.

which are most likely to arrest his attention. The signs, also, vary very much in the same person.

As the paroxysm approaches, the patient may become unusually fidgety, or irritable, or moody, or forgetful, or absent, or drowsy. Or he may sleep restlessly, grinding his teeth, snoring or snorting, dreaming about things which distress or terrify him, or even walking while asleep. Or he may have a disagreeable feeling of tightness about the throat, with cramps and tinglings in the limbs and elsewhere. Or he may be unusually "shaky," and now and then, as in a patient at present under my care, he may be annoyed with frequent shudderings of a very disagreeable and violent character.

Another sign of danger may be giddiness or headache, but so far as the latter symptom is concerned, I should not be disposed to lay much stress upon it as a warning in simple epilepsy.

Occasionally, the pupils may be more dilated and sluggish than usual, or one pupil may be more dilated and sluggish than the other, or the eyes may be rotated in a peculiar manner.

Usually, so far as my own experience goes, the pulse may become feebler than it was before; and not unfrequently the patient will complain that nothing will warm him or keep him warm, or else he may sigh in a way which shows that he is not breathing so freely as he ought to do.

Later still, there may be certain vague and undefinable sensations or movements, very varying in their character, but all comprehended under the name *aura*—sensations of pain, numbness, tingling, or a feeling as of cold vapour; movements of shuddering or spasm—beginning in a distant part, as in the hand or foot, and travelling towards the head. In other words, there may be certain symptoms which, as Dr. Watson thinks, are in some degree analogous to those of *globus* in hysteria, or to the numb and tingling feelings which are the frequent precursors of paralysis and apoplexy.

In some cases there may be a special premonition. In one of my patients, the fit is invariably preceded by an intense feeling of hunger. In another patient, since insane, a little blue imp perched upon the table, and moped and mocked at him as he lost his consciousness. In a third, a guitar seemed to have been roughly grated near the ear. But these signs are of little value, for they are only perceptible to the patient, and not even to him until he has ceased to be able to bestir himself.

Last of all, there is a sign which is very difficult to catch, and this is the death-like pallor which overspreads the countenance immediately before the fall. M. Trousseau called attention to this sign, in a recent lecture at the Hôtel Dieu, in Paris,[1] as one

[1] L'Union Médicale, 28th April, 1855.

which is diagnostic of epilepsy; and since this time I have seen it in all the instances, now amounting to twenty-one, in which I have seen the fit from the very beginning. "Il est une signe," says M. Trousseau, "qui se produit au moment de la chute, et qui n'est imitable pour personne, c'est la pâleur très prononcée, cadavérique, qui couvre pour un instant la face de l'épileptique; nous ne la voyons pas, parceque nous arrivons toujours trop tard, alors que la face est dejà d'un rouge très prononcé." M. Delasiauve has also noticed the same phenomenon in many cases.[1]

—In the severest and most characteristic form of the paroxysm, the patient utters a peculiar cry, and at once falls down convulsed and insensible, or he falls without making any noise at all. The convulsions are usually more marked on one side of the body than the other. They drag the mouth towards the side which is most affected, and twist the face in the opposite direction until the chin may rest upon the shoulder. They push forward the tongue and clench the teeth upon it. They clasp the thumb upon the palm, and hold it there with a force which seems to be more than muscular. They seize the walls of the chest and abdomen, and put an end to the movements of respiration. They

[1] Traité de l'Epilepsie, 8vo, Paris, 1854.

stiffen the limbs so as to make it very difficult to bend them. In some instances they may take hold of the bladder, or bowel, or seminal vesicles, and expel the contents; in others, they may be so violent as to bite off a large portion of the tongue, or break the teeth, or dislocate a limb. At first it seems as if the muscles would never relax, but afterwards the contractions are separated by intervals which grow wider as the paroxysm draws to an end. The convulsions, that is to say, are tetanoid at first, clonic afterwards.

At the instant of the fall, a corpse-like paleness overspreads the countenance; a few instants later, and the whole appearance suggests the idea of a person struggling under the bowstring of some invisible executioner, for the original paleness rapidly changes into livid blueness, or even blackness, the head and neck become frightfully bloated, and there are hissing, gurgling, choking sounds in the throat, which show very clearly that the patient is in the actual throes of suffocation. At times, however, the signs of suffocation are absent, and the ghastly paleness of the beginning is retained throughout.

When the fit is at its height, a quantity of frothy saliva is usually blown or puffed from the mouth; and if the tongue or cheek has been bitten, this saliva is not unfrequently reddened with blood.

If the eyelids are open, the eye is seen to be projected and distorted, with its pupil dilated to the utmost, and absolutely insensible to light. As a rule, however, the eyelids would seem to be closed, and well it is that they are so, for it requires some nerve to meet the hideous stare of the epileptic eye.

All this while it is usual for the hands and feet to be cool, and bedewed with clammy perspiration. Except the head and neck, indeed, the whole body is cooler than natural; and if the head and neck are warmer than the rest, it is merely because their vessels are more distended with venous blood.

The other and less obvious features of the paroxysm are in keeping with these.

At first, the pulse may be almost silent, and the action of the heart very feeble: but if the finger be kept upon the wrist and the hand placed upon the bosom, it is found that the pulse may rapidly acquire a force and fulness which it never had in the intervals between the fits, and that the heart may beat tumultuously and with great violence as the pulse rises. In some instances, however, the pulse may remain almost silent, and the action of the heart extremely feeble, from beginning to end.

From the very first all consciousness is happily suspended—this is our only consolation in so sad a spectacle—and the most powerful stimulants fail to evoke any sign of action in the dormant mind. The water which may be poured upon the face (with few exceptions) causes no blinking in the open and staring eye; or the fire upon which the patient has fallen may char the flesh without causing a single pang.

After continuing for two or three minutes, which seem drawn out to hours, the convulsions cease, and the patient is left with all his muscles unstrung, like a person dead drunk, or struck down by apoplexy. The lungs, no longer restrained by the suffocative spasm of the earlier part of the fit, resume their play with a deep inspiration, and then act with loud and stertorous breathings; and as they do this, the veins of the head and neck become unloaded, the natural colour returns to the surface, and the pulse to the arteries, and last of all, the patient wakes to an obscured and troubled consciousness. His first feelings are those of surprise and fatigue; his first words are expressive of suffering. "Je suis brisé," Calmeil tells us, were often the first words of the returning epileptic at the Salpêtrière or Charenton. The time during which the patient lies after a fit before awaking is very variable, but it is rarely more than half an hour, and it may not be more than two or three minutes.

This is the usual, but not the invariable course of the fit. Indeed, the attempts at rallying may be very imperfect, and fit after fit may recur for a long period without any interval of waking, or all rallying may be prevented by death.

— After waking there are generally some symptoms of reaction in the circulation; but in simple epilepsy these are never very marked. They may be enough to give a dull flush to the cheek and a little fulness to the pulse, for a short time after the patient wakes; but, as a rule, these symptoms cease when the coma ceases, and the coma is never much prolonged in simple epilepsy. Usually the patient is headachy and exhausted, listless and stunned, moody and irritable, until a night's rest has enabled him to recover the balance of his shaken nervous system. The jaded countenance also tells plainly of the past struggle, even though it may present none of those numerous and minute dots of ecchymosis about the eyelids and upon the forehead, which are such unequivocal signs of a severe attack of epilepsy.

As time goes on the mental faculties recover more and more imperfectly, and more and more tardily, and at last their habitual state may be one of pitiful fatuity, from which no single ray of the Divine principle beams forth. Or the moodiness and irritability which follow the attack may become more and more marked, until at last they merge into attacks of downright mania. Or symptoms of paralysis may make their appearance. Or death may happen in a fit or shortly afterwards. The natural tendency of epilepsy is assuredly towards dementia; and dementia is the final doom of the epileptic, if his disorder be unchecked and life prolonged sufficiently; and this equally, whether symptoms of insanity have or have not been developed; but at the same time, it is possible for an epileptic to have many fits and live many years, without ever losing the powers which are necessary to render him an agreeable and serviceable member of society. If death happens, it happens most generally from exhaustion in the period of prostration immediately following the paroxysm.

— But though always cheerless, the picture of epilepsy is not always so dark and gloomy as is here depicted, and in some instances the several features may be so softened down, as to be recognised with difficulty.

In the slightest form of the malady, the patient pauses suddenly in the midst of anything he may happen to be doing or saying at the time, his countenance becomes pale and blank, his lungs cease to play, and, after a momentary feeling of giddiness or absence, he is himself again. His memory has kept no record of this sad passage in his history, and if it had escaped the notice of others, he might never know anything about it. Or, in addition to these symptoms, a lurid flush may succeed to the paleness of the countenance, the veins of the neck and forehead may stand out in more prominent relief, the face may turn towards one of the shoulders, and there may be some convulsive twitching in the face and neck, and arm or arms. In such a case there is no scream or cry, no fall, no bitten tongue, no foam at the mouth, and at most there is only some obscure gurgling in the throat, some staggering, and some slight moistening of the lips with saliva. In such a case the convulsive movements are very partial, rarely extending beyond the face, neck, or arm, but in some few instances the whole frame may be agitated by one or two violent convulsive shocks. This state of giddiness and absence and partial spasm, may be followed by more or less fatigue, or loss of memory, or confusion of thought, or depression of spirits, or irritability of temper, and at times it may end in positive drowsiness or actual sleep; but usually recovery is almost instantaneous.

In some of these cases, moreover, it would seem, not only that the patient does not fall or cry, or suffer from general convulsion, but that the state of intellectual eclipse — the most characteristic symptom of epilepsy — is far from complete. Esquirol says, "il est des accès dans lesquels on n'observe pas la perte de connaissance;" and M. Herpin directs particular attention to such cases.

These cases, however, are very rare, or at any rate they are very difficult to detect, if other proof be wanted than the mere assurance of the patient. They are common enough in certain chronic diseases of the brain, as meningitis or tumour, but in simple epilepsy they would seem to be extremely rare. Cases, however, are on record, and the following, which fell under my own notice, may perhaps be added to the number.

CASE.—This patient, Mr. P—, æt. 18, was the son of a farmer living near Leicester. Early in the summer of 1855, he suffered from unusual palpitations upon any exertion, and later in the same year he had frequent fits, such as will be presently described. He had been growing rapidly, and in addition to this he had imprudently exposed himself to the sun while out in the fields during harvest. These attacks occurred at frequent intervals until the beginning of May, 1857, when one night he had a severe fit, in which there was convulsion and bitten tongue.

Mr. P— came to see me on the 21st May, 1857, and at that time I found him to be a tall, over-grown lad, with a dilated and sluggish pupil, a weak, slow pulse (60), and a curiously shaped head, evidently not bright, but without any positive signs of mental deficiency. I had just noticed these points, and my finger was still on his pulse, when he told me that he was going to have a fit; and upon looking up, I saw that his features had become pale and drawn, his eyes fixed, his lips slightly moistened with saliva, and his face already turned round to the right shoulder. I also heard certain choking sounds in the throat. On placing my hands on each side of the chest, I found that the respiratory movements were altogether at an end. These symptoms continued for a sufficient time to allow a lurid flush to take the place of the original paleness of the countenance, and then, drawing a deep sigh, he suddenly recovered. His pulse at the beginning of the attack was 60, and very weak; after the attack it rose to 80, became fuller, and the heart throbbed a little. On returning to himself, he stated spontaneously that his vision was troubled in the attack, and that he had heard a remark which I had made to his mother, who was with him. He also told me that such attacks occurred several times a day, and that he never lost his consciousness in them.

I saw Mr. P— again on the 1st of November, 1857, and on this occasion I had another opportunity of witnessing an attack. In this attack, as in the one just described, the face was first pale then lurid, the features were drawn, the eyes fixed, the lips moistened with a little saliva, the face twisted round to the right shoulder, the chest immoveable, and choking sounds proceeded from the throat; and in addition to these symptoms, the right arm was rigidly contracted and agitated by slight convulsive shocks, and both hands had seized tight hold of the arms of the chair in which he was sitting. Wishing on this occasion to test the condition of the consciousness, I pinched his hand, and asked him if he felt pain. He moved his head a little, and there was an expression in his eye and a motion in his lip, which appeared to indicate a wish to speak. I then held my watch before his face, and as I did this, he began, as it seemed, to try to overcome the spasm which had twisted his head round, and in a moment or two succeeded. On returning to himself, he said that he had made several voluntary attempts to overcome the spasm which had turned his head round to the side, and that he always did this if the fit continued longer than usual; and on asking what I had done during the attack, he told me, without the least prompting on my part, that I had pinched his hand and held my watch before his face, or what he supposed to be my watch, for, as in the former instance, his vision was greatly troubled. After the attack his countenance had a flushed and jaded expression.

I have seen Mr. P— once since the last date, and witnessed another attack of the same nature, only less marked than the two which have been described. I also learn that he has had a repetition of the severer form of attack on more than one occasion.

3. *Of the appearances after death in epilepsy.*

The morbid appearances after death from *simple epilepsy* are necessarily more than obscure, if the case have really been one of simple epilepsy. In cases fatal during the fit the brain has been found to be congested; but this appearance is clearly owing to the manner of death, and it is allowed to be so. In cases, again, where epilepsy has been complicated with insanity, the brain or its membranes may present various signs of inflammation, or of changes more or less akin to inflammation; but these signs are clearly referrible to the mental disorder, and this for no other reason than that they are as common, or more common, in insanity without epilepsy than in insanity with epilepsy. In other cases there are signs of degeneracy, such as pallor of the grey matter, softening, induration, atrophy, dropsical effusion, but these are the very signs which belong to the demented state. It is this very fact, however, which furnishes some grounds for supposing that signs of this character may have something to do with epilepsy. It does so, because the demented state is intimately connected with convulsive disorder; for if a demented person be not epileptic, he is almost sure to be afflicted with palsied shakings, or cramps, or spasms, in one form or another. In other cases, again, the skull may be thicker and heavier than usual, and the several internal projections, as the clinoid processes, may be considerably developed, or various portions of the dura mater may be converted into bone. Such changes, however, though common, are by no means constant. Indeed, there are no constant changes —not even that change in the pituitary body, of which so much was said by Wenzel, for speaking respecting it, Rokitansky says that he has "frequently failed to discover it in those who had notoriously suffered from epilepsy and convulsions;" and that he has "met with it in others who had been thoroughly healthy." It will be necessary, however, to speak more particularly of these changes when speaking of epileptiform convulsions. Indeed, I have no proper right to refer to them now, for if epilepsy can be referred to any one of the affections which have been mentioned, then it ceases to be simple epilepsy, and becomes an epileptiform affection arising from such and such a disease. At the same time these remarks, though somewhat out of place, are expedient, as showing in an indirect manner that epilepsy is not connected with an overactive state of brain.

4. *Of the pathology of epilepsy.*

(*a.*) *Of the pathology as deduced from a consideration of the phenomena connected with the vascular system.*

The frigid and clammy hand, the foot that will scarcely keep warm before the fire, the pale and sallow or dark and venous complexion, the habitual feeling of chilliness, are facts which appear to show that the circulation is wanting in vigour; and this inference is fully borne out by the pulse, which in simple epilepsy is rarely otherwise than weak and slow. Plethora, in the form so often exhibited in the butcher, is never met with, and feverish reaction is a rare occurrence, even as an accident. There are, indeed, cases of *epileptiform* disease, in which the circulation may exhibit a greater degree of activity, but these cases, as will be seen in the proper place, present no real objection to the conclusion that the habitual state of the circulation in epilepsy is one of depression.

Nor is there any evidence of a contrary character in the fit itself. Upon the eve of the fit, if any change can be perceived, it is in all probability one in which the skin has become paler and more dusky than usual, and the pulse more feeble. At the instant of the fall, in many, if not in all instances, a corpse-like pallor overspreads the countenance—a phenomenon which can only be explained on the supposition that syncope is impending; a moment or two afterwards, a dull-red flush, rapidly deepening into livid blueness, or even blackness, takes the place of the paleness which had first overspread the countenance, the face and neck become frightfully bloated, and everything shows plainly that all respiration is at an end. This state of suffocation continues during the whole course of the convulsion, and so perfect is it, that little or no arterial blood can find its way into the arteries during the convulsion.

There is, however, one fact which may be thought to show that there is an increased injection of arterial blood into the vessels during the convulsion. Such injection is evidently very imperfect at the onset of the fit—in many instances at least, for upon no other supposition can we explain the corpse-like paleness of the countenance, and the feeble and silent pulse at the wrist. This is evident. But if the finger be kept upon the wrist, it may be found that the pulse may rise during the convulsion, until it has acquired a force and fulness which it never had in the intervals between the fits; and if the hand be placed over the heart at this time, it may be found that this organ is beating tumultuously and with great violence. It may also be found that these signs of vascular excitement will continue for some time after the convulsion is over. These facts are evident and unmistakeable, but they do not show, as they might seem to do at first sight, that more *arterial* blood is injected into the arteries at this time. On the contrary, they necessitate a totally different conclusion when they are subjected to a strict scrutiny.

Now it cannot be doubted, that the effect of cutting off the access of air to the blood is to prevent the free passage of the blood through the pulmonary capillaries, and to overload the right side of the heart and the venous system generally, at the expense of the left side of the heart and the arteries springing from it. In this way the right side of the heart may become so much distended that the auriculo-ventricular valves are separated, and the beatings of the ventricle are made to tell as much in driving the blood back into the veins, as in sending it onwards into the lungs. But it is not right to suppose that the arteries are empty. If, for example, the carotid of a rabbit be exposed, and a ligature placed around the windpipe, it is found that the blood continues to flow through the vessel, that the originally scarlet colour becomes darker and darker, until at last it is as black as that of the blood in the neighbouring jugulars. Two minutes to two minutes and a half are occupied in this transformation of the scarlet into black blood. It is found, also, that this black blood will escape from the cut vessel in as full a stream and with as much force at the expiration of two minutes or two minutes and a half from the commencement of the process of suffocation, as it did before the aëration of the blood was at all interfered with. Nay, it is even found that at this time the black blood will escape with greater force and in a fuller stream than it did when it was red, for on fitting a hæmadynometer into the vessel and testing the force of the pulse-wave before and after the tightening of the ligature upon the windpipe, the mercury in the instrument is seen to rise to a higher point than that to which it rose previously. Indeed, at this time it is evident, without the aid of any instrument, that the artery is more distended and more tense than it was before. This phenomenon is explained by the late Professor John Reid, who has investigated the condition of the circulation in suffocation more carefully and successfully than any other observer,[1] as the result of an impediment to the free passage of the black blood through the systemic capillaries similar to that which prevents the free

[1] 'Phys., Anat., and Pathol. Researches,' 8vo, Edinb. 1848.

passage of the same blood through the pulmonic capillaries, and it is more easy to entertain this view, and to suppose that, in consequence of this impediment in the systemic capillaries, a greater proportion of the force of the left ventricle is expended in distending the arteries, than to suppose that the ventricle is "stimulated" to increased action under these circumstances. And, lastly, as explaining the peculiarity of the pulse in suffocation, it is to be remembered that the blood is sent along the arteries with greater force and increased velocity during violent attempts at *expiration,* and that the pulse becomes soft, feeble, and less frequent during violent attempts at *inspiration;* and hence it may be supposed that the increased fulness and force of the pulse during the suffocation of epilepsy may be owing partly to the fact that during the whole of this time the air is prevented from entering the chest by the firm spasm of all the muscles concerned—a state which may be compared to that which obtains in forced and prolonged expiration.

Hence, the increase in the strength and fulness of the pulse which may take place during the convulsion of epilepsy is no proof, as it might appear at first sight, that the brain as well as the rest of the system is at this time supplied with an increased quantity of arterial blood, for the black and bloated face and neck, and the absolute suspension of the respiratory movements, shew most clearly that the pulse is then filled, not with red blood, but with black.

After the convulsion there is little to notice in the circulation. When the convulsions cease the respiration is speedily restored, and the readmission of arterial blood into the system may be attended with some transitory and inconsiderable febrile reaction; but this reaction has nothing whatever to do with the convulsion, for when it appears the convulsion has departed, and if the convulsion returns it is not until the reaction has first taken its departure.

Arguing, therefore, from the corpse-like paleness and comparative pulselessness of the onset of the paroxysm, and from the signs of positive and unmistakeable suffocation by which this stage of paleness and pulselessness is succeeded, the only conclusion would seem to be that the convulsion of epilepsy is connected with the want of a due supply of arterial blood. Indeed, the whole history of the paroxysm, as deduced from the condition of the vascular system, would seem to show that there is something utterly uncongenial between epilepsy and anything like arterial excitement.

Nor is it any objection to this view, that the convulsion ceases when the blood has become thoroughly deprived of its arterial properties. On the contrary, the cessation of the convulsion at this time *may* be easily explained as the natural effect of the way in which the *nerves* must suffer from this very want of arterial blood. At any rate, it is certain that the nerves cannot discharge their office of conductors unless they are supplied with a due quantity of arterial blood. If, for example, the circulation in the hand be depressed or suspended by immersing the part in iced water, the power of feeling and of throwing the muscles into action, whether voluntarily or involuntarily, is partially or wholly destroyed. If the principal vessel of a limb be tied a similar result ensues, until the collateral circulation is established. And hence it may be assumed, that there is a point in the process of suffocation, where, wanting the due supply of arterial blood, the nerves will cease to be conductors, and where, consequently, the convulsions will come to an end,—for, upon any hypothesis, it is evident that the convulsions will come to an end when the muscles are no longer required to respond to that change in the nervous centres which is concerned in producing contraction in the muscles.

— But, it may be asked, is there no change in the blood itself? Is there not some important truth in the " humoral theory of epilepsy," as recently advanced by Dr. Todd? " I hold," says this distinguished physician, " that the peculiar features of an epileptic seizure are due to the gradual accumulation of a morbid material in the blood, until it reaches such an amount that it operates upon the brain in, as it were, an explosive manner; in other words, the influence of this morbid matter, when in sufficient quantity, excites a highly polarized state of the brain, or of certain parts of it, and these discharge their nervous power upon certain other parts of the cerebro-spinal centre in such a way as to give rise to the phenomena of the fit. A very analogous effect is that which results from the administration of strychnia, which is best seen in a cold-blooded animal, like the frog. You may administer this drug in very minute quantities for some time, without producing any sensible effect; but when the quantity has accumulated in the system up to a certain point, then the smallest increase of dose will immediately give rise to the peculiar convulsive phenomena. This is the humoral theory of epilepsy. It assumes that the essential derangement of health consists in the generation of a morbid matter, which infects the blood; and it supposes that this morbid matter has a special affinity for the brain, or for certain parts of it, as the strychnia, in the case just cited, exercises a special affinity for the spinal cord. The source of this morbid matter is probably in the nervous system, it may be in the brain itself. It may owe its origin to a disturbed nutrition—an imperfect secondary assimilation of that organ—and in its turn it will create additional disturbance in the functions and the nutrition of the brain. Probably, in no instance does an epileptic fit ever occur without leaving a damaged state of brain, which in some cases is permanent, in others remarkably transient." And again: "According to the humoral theory, the variety in the nature and severity of the fits depends on the quantity of the poisonous or morbid material, and on the part of the brain which it chiefly or primarily affects. If it affect primarily the hemispheres, and spend itself, as it were, on them alone, you have only the epileptic vertigo. If it affect primarily the region of the quadrigeminal bodies, or if the affection of the hemispheres extend to that region, then you will have the epileptic fit fully developed."[1]

This theory is based upon the well-known connexion between the presence of urea in the blood (or carbonate of ammonia resulting from the decomposition of urea)—the result of defective renal action—and the epileptic condition; and it might also have been based upon the connexion between convulsion and blood over-loaded with bile. But if there be any evidence in these facts in favour of the existence of this hypothetical morbid material, there is none in favour of the idea that its *modus*

[1] 'Med. Times and Gaz.,' 5th and 12th August, 1854.

operandi is by exciting a highly polarized state of the brain, if by this state is meant anything like a condition of excitement. On the contrary, it is certain (as will be shown eventually) that the action of the brain, and of the nervous system generally, is reduced almost to zero at the time when convulsion is brought about by the accumulation of urea or bile in the blood; and it is more than probable, that strychnia, instead of acting as Dr. Todd supposes it to act—that is, by exciting a highly polarized state of some part of nervous system—acts (p. 91) by reducing the stimulating powers of the blood, and by diminishing the irritability of the nerves and muscles.

There is no difficulty, however, in believing that retained excretions may play an important part in the production of disease, and of epilepsy among the rest. Indeed, it is scarcely to be doubted that a free discharge in the office of excretion, not only in the kidney and liver, but in every other excretory organ, is essential to the existence of healthy blood; and it may well be believed that an imperfect discharge of the office of excretion *in one or other of the excretory organs* may lead to the accumulation of effete matter in the blood, and that this accumulation of effete matter may be a not unimportant cause in bringing about an attack of epilepsy. But there is no manner of reason for supposing that the blood under these circumstances becomes more stimulating. On the contrary, the conclusion which arises out of the history of cases where the urine or bile is suppressed is the natural conclusion, and this is, that blood thus altered is less fit to discharge its several offices, or, in other words, less stimulating.

— It would seem, then, that the phenomena connected with the vascular system are altogether opposed to the idea of arterial excitement in epilepsy. It would seem, indeed, as if the spasms, as well as the loss of consciousness and sensibility, were connected with a deficiency of arterial blood, for in the first place, there is a state closely approaching to syncope, and in the next place, a state of positive suffocation, or arrested arterialization of the blood. It is not improbable, also, that the blood may have been previously rendered less stimulating than it ought to be by the imperfect exercise of some organ of excretion. The phenomena, indeed, are in harmony with the previous considerations respecting muscular action, for, according to them, the office of the blood is to antagonize contraction, not to cause it.

Nor does there appear to be any reason for supposing that venous congestion has a more important part to play in the production of epilepsy than that which has been assigned to arterial injection. No doubt the veins of the brain and head generally are congested from a very early moment, but there is a moment antecedent to this in which the death-like paleness of the face—in many cases at least—is a sufficient proof that the veins were emptier than usual before they became congested. Indeed, it may be supposed that this was the case in the majority of instances, if not in all, for there would seem to be no way of accounting for the instantaneous loss of consciousness and sensibility (which is in reality the first phenomenon of the fit), except upon the supposition of some sudden failure in the supply of blood to the great nervous centres. At any rate, the well-known anatomical difficulty is not the sole difficulty which has to be overcome before it can be supposed that Dr. Marshall Hall's hypothesis of *trachelismus*—or the prevention of the return of blood from the brain by the spasm of certain muscles in the neck—has anything to do with the causation of epilepsy.

(*b.*) *The pathology of epilepsy as deduced from a consideration of the phenomena connected with the nervous system.*

Interrogating the nervous system from a mental point of view, the facts will scarcely warrant the idea that epilepsy is connected with anything like over-action of the nervous system. On the contrary, everything seems to point to a state which is the very opposite of this. Thus, the want of memory, the want of intelligence, the want of fancy, the want of purpose, which are habitual; the utter annihilation of everything mental in the fit itself; and the gloom and prostration which remain after the fit; all go to confirm the impression of mental inaction which is so generally conveyed at the very first glance by the dilated and sluggish pupil, and by the torpid features.

Nor is a contrary opinion to be drawn from the fact, that epilepsy is frequently connected with insanity—so frequently, that out of 339 epileptics whose histories were analysed by Esquirol, 269, or four fifths, were also insane—for out of these cases of double disorder, the greater part by far were persons whose mental state was the negation of everything active. And in the remaining few, whose derangement may be supposed to have been of a more active complexion, it does not follow that the convulsion was directly connected with any state of mental excitement. On the contrary, it will be allowed by all those who are practically acquainted with these deplorable cases, that the time for the convulsion is the period of collapse following the excitement and receiving the first shadows of that mental eclipse which is about to be.

It would seem also that no different conclusion

can be drawn from the morbid appearances which are presented after death. If these chance to indicate previous inflammation, it does not follow that the convulsion had anything to do with the inflammation as an active process, for it may have been connected with a prior or subsequent period of exhaustion. Indeed, the history of *epileptiform* convulsion, as will appear presently, shows most conclusively, that the convulsion is connected with one or other of these periods of exhaustion, and not with the period of inflammatory excitement. And surely it is not possible to draw any other conclusion from the appearances which are common to epilepsy and dementia—the pallor of the grey substance, the atrophy, the chronic softening and induration, the dropsical effusion, and the rest. Is it possible for such conditions to indicate anything but a state of brain which is the reverse of everything active? And certainly, the thickened skull, or an ossified or cartilaginous condition of certain parts of the dura mater, is no argument in favour of over-action of the brain. On the contrary, it may be supposed, without any undue stretch of fancy, that this excess of ossification *may* indicate vital degradation, for bone holds a low grade among the tissues, and in this way the excess of bone may be a sort of argument that the neighbouring brain is wanting in vital energy.

During the convulsion the state of the brain is one of coma. During the convulsion, that is to say, the state of the brain, regarded mentally, is one of extremest inaction.

It would seem also that the brain cannot be active in any sense under these circumstances; for if, as there is every reason to believe, the brain obeys the law under which all other organs are placed, and requires a due supply of arterial blood as the condition of its action, then must the action be reduced to zero, when, as in the fit of epilepsy, the state of the circulation is first of all closely akin to syncope, and afterwards one of complete suffocation, or arrested arterialization of the blood. Indeed, it would seem to be as impossible for the action of the brain to continue in epilepsy as in the well-known experiment by Sir Astley Cooper, in which epileptiform convulsion is caused by tying the carotids and compressing the vertebrals—an experiment which might almost of itself serve as the key to the interpretation of convulsion. "I tied," says Sir Astley, "the carotid arteries of a rabbit. Respiration was somewhat quickened, and the heart's action increased, but no other effect was produced. In five minutes the vertebral arteries were compressed by the thumbs, the trachea being completely excluded. Respiration almost directly stopped, convulsive struggles succeeded;

the animal lost its consciousness, and appeared dead. The pressure was removed, and it recovered with a convulsive inspiration. It laid upon its side making violent convulsive efforts, breathed laboriously, and its heart beat rapidly. In two hours it had recovered, but its respiration was laborious. The vertebrals were compressed a second time. Respiration stopped; then succeeded convulsive struggles, loss of motion, and apparent death. When let loose, its natural functions returned with a loud inspiration, and with breathing excessively laboured. In four hours it was moving about, and ate some greens. In five hours the vertebral arteries were compressed a third time, and with the same effect. In seven hours it was cleaning its face with its paw. In nine hours the vertebral arteries were compressed for the fifth time, and the result was the same; namely, suspended respiration, convulsions, loss of motion and consciousness. On the removal of pressure, violent and laborious respirations ensued, and afterwards the breathing became very quick. After forty-eight hours, for the sixth time, the compression was applied with the same effect."[1]

Nor is it easy to understand how the medulla

---

[1] Some experiments and observations on tying the Carotid and Vertebral Arteries, &c. 'Guy's Hospital Reports,' No. 3, p. 465, Sept. 1836.

oblongata, the spinal cord, or any other nervous centre can be in a different case to the brain; for, upon the same principles of reasoning, these centres are sources of innervation just in proportion to the activity of the arterial circulation in them. Indeed, if arterial blood in proper quantity is necessary to the generation of "nervous influence," then must this generation be almost, if not altogether, nil at the time when the muscles strain under the convulsions of epilepsy.

But is there nothing else? Is there no peculiar state of the nervous system in epilepsy? Is there no *morbid irritability?* In order to answer this question it is necessary to ask another—What is morbid irritability? It is not inflammation, it is not fever; it is some indefinable and negative state which frequently occurs in teething, in worm disease, in uterine derangement, and in many other cases; a state in which the patient is unusually depressed by depressing influences, and unusually excited by exciting influences. But what is this state? Is it anything more than mere exhaustion? In difficult teething the strength is worn away by pain and want of sleep; in worm-disease the system is starved and exhausted by its hungry parasites; in uterine derangement the health is undermined, in all probability, by pain, or by sanguineous and other discharges. In each case there is unequivocal exhaustion of body and mind, and the symptoms of morbid irritability appear to be no other than the signs of such exhaustion. A weak person is more affected by the several agencies which act upon the body, because he has lost some of that innate strength which belongs to the strong person; and a person who is morbidly irritable, is in reality one who, for want of this principle of strength, responds impatiently to the several stimuli which are appointed to call out his vital phenomena. In a word, this undue morbid irritability may be nothing else than the natural consequence of that general state of exhaustion, the signs of which are so legibly written upon the vascular and nervous systems of the epileptic. Indeed, after what has been said in the physiological premises, this is the only conclusion.

For what, according to these premises, is the *modus operandi* of irritation? It is (pp. 79—88) no other than this—that irritation, however brought about, acts by exhausting, and not by stimulating, the nerve and muscle.

And what, according to the same premises, is the significance of morbid irritability—of a state, that is to say, in which the muscles are more apt to contract when irritated, and more prone to remain contracted when contracted? It is not that these muscles are more supplied with nervous influence. It is (pp. 62—64) that they are less supplied with this influence. Thus, the muscles of the two hind legs of a frog become more irritable when the influence proceeding from the brain is cut off from them by dividing the spinal cord; and the muscles of one of these legs are rendered more irritable than the muscles of the other when they are cut off from the spinal cord by dividing the nerves where they leave the spinal column. It would seem, indeed, as if the disposition to muscular contraction were most antagonized where the largest amount of nervous influence was supplied to the muscles.

There is no necessity, then, to look upon this morbid state of irritability as an evidence of the existence of any peculiar condition in some part of the nervous system; for, thus interpreted, it only signifies a state in which the muscles are ill supplied with nervous influence. Thus interpreted, indeed, morbid irritability only becomes another name for inefficient action of the nervous system.

— The pathology of epilepsy, therefore, as deduced from a consideration of the phenomena belonging to the nervous system is in harmony with what had been already deduced from a consideration of the phenomena belonging to the vascular system, and the conclusion is precisely what was to be expected from the previous investigations respecting the physiology of muscular action.

From these previous investigations it was to be expected that coma and convulsion might go hand in hand together—for muscular contraction, according to these investigations, is to be looked for when a failure in the action of the nervous centres causes a failure in the amount of "nervous influence" distributed to the muscles; and thus, this difficulty of the association of coma and convulsion being at an end, we need no longer repeat the questions which Foville asks despairingly—" Pourquoi tandis que l'intelligence et la sensibilité sont complètement abolies, l'action musculaire est elle si souvent partée au plus haut degré d'intensité qu'elle puisse atteindre ? Pourquoi cette opposition si tranchée dans deux ordres de symptômes fournis par la souffrance du même organe ? Comment se peut-il que la même altération survenue brusquement paralyse l'intelligence et la sensibilité, et excite au plus haut degré l'action des muscles ? En d'autres termes, pourquoi, par suite d'un dérangement subitement développé, la portion des centres nerveux qui préside à l'intelligence et à la sensibilité est-elle anéantie dans son action, tandis que celle qui préside aux mouvemens voluntaires se trouve assez violemment excitée pour produire d'horribles convulsions ?"

5. *Of the treatment of epilepsy.*

Arguing from the physiological and pathological premises, it may be inferred that epilepsy will have to be cured by strengthening and stimulating the system, and not by debilitating or depressing it; and this inference is not altogether at variance with experience. On the contrary, the growing disposition to leave nature to her own course, and the growing dissatisfaction with all "lowering measures," may be accepted as a strong argument against the opinion that epileptics have been really benefited by these measures. The necessity for a tonic and stimulating plan of treatment, however, does not rest merely upon *à priori* inferences, or upon the unsatisfactory results of an opposite kind of practice; and this will appear in due time.

(1. It is not necessary to suppose that epileptics are injured by a liberal diet. On the contrary, the full allowance of good substantial food is given to the epileptics who are cared for in our county lunatic asylums, and in some of these establishments it is the rule to treat them more liberally than the other inmates. For my own part I am in the habit of recommending a liberal diet, in which there is no stint of animal food, and cer-

tainly I know of no disadvantages from such a course. Indeed, I have often seen unquestionable signs of benefit from such a diet, particularly in cases where a patient has been for some time upon an opposite course. Nor does there appear to be much reason for supposing that epileptics are often troubled with difficulty of digestion. There are occasions, no doubt, in which their stomach misbehaves a little, but these occasions are apt to occur more frequently when it is supposed that the patient cannot eat this or cannot eat that, than when he is allowed to have a fair amount of that licence in matters of eating which is conceded to others. Quantity, I take it, is of far greater importance than quality, and if, on the one hand, care be taken never to overload the stomach with more food than it can conveniently dispose of, and, on the other hand, never to leave the stomach empty for too long a time, it really does not seem to matter much what is eaten. Indeed, I have never found it necessary to disturb the arrangements of a household by requiring an epileptic to be fed differently to the rest of the family.

Nor is the prejudice against the use of stimulants founded on any better reason. Beer, indeed, is given to epileptics in many lunatic asylums, and, to say the least, no harm is found to result from the practice. Beer and wine are also allowed in not a few instances under ordinary circumstances, and in many, not only without any harm, but with apparent benefit. For my own part I am in the constant habit of recommending a liberal allowance of stimulants, and certainly I have seen nothing yet to make me at all doubtful of the propriety of this course. I have, indeed, notes of four cases in which patients who had before objected to the use of wine or beer from conscientious scruples, only began to improve when they had been induced to alter their habits in this respect; and on more than one occasion a patient has told me that he had succeeded in warding off a fit by a glass of wine. Indeed, so satisfied am I of the beneficial effects of stimulants, that I should not be very sanguine about the recovery of a patient who could not obtain them, or would not use them.

In keeping with these considerations it would seem that epileptics are more benefited by coffee, which is a potent stimulant, than by tea, which is rather a sedative. That coffee is a potent stimulant there can be little doubt. The student takes it to keep himself awake and warm. The opium-eater takes it to enhance the stimulating effects of the opium, or to dispel the subsequent drowsiness; and it is given to him if he has overdosed himself. The inhabitants of hot countries trust to it for dispelling languor and lassitude, and it does not disappoint them. The Arabs find it indispensable in their long rides across the weary desert. "The hunters of the Isle of France and Bourbon," says Southey,[1] "take no other provision into the wood; and Bruce tells us that the viaticum of the Gallas in their expeditions consists of balls of ground coffee and butter; one per diem, the size of a walnut, sufficing to prevent the sense of fatigue." Tea, on the other hand, seems to exert a sedative influence after the heating effects of the hot water in which it is infused have passed off. Be the explanation what it may, however, I have satisfied myself by oft-repeated trials, that epileptics can take coffee with positive advantage almost at any time, and that they are often rendered much more "nervous" by the use of tea, particularly at an early period in the day.

In any case there is no question as to the necessity of ordering the habits in such a way as to save the strength as much as possible. There is no question as to the advisability of continence in sexual matters. There is no question as to the inadvisability of taxing the brain with severe study. But there may be a question as to the correctness of the rule which is usually laid down with regard to bodily exercise. Arguing from the premises, there would seem to be no ground for supposing

[1] 'Correspondence,' vol. iv, p. 300.

that the epileptic had any spare energy which must be worked down by exercise, and so far this idea is fully confirmed by experience. More than once I have found a patient begin to improve when he became careful to avoid muscular fatigue; more than once I have known a patient begin to retrograde, who began to try his strength too speedily. Not long ago I had a note from a medical gentleman, in which he told me that a patient about whom he had consulted me, had gone on very well so long as he had carried out an order which required him to ride to and from his place of business in the city, and that the fits had returned with their accustomed frequency after he had begun disregard this order.

2. The ordinary way of treating epilepsy at the present day is very different to what it was when almost all disorders were referred to inflammation, or over-action of one kind or another. It is now no longer the habit to bleed either by the lancet or by leeches. It is now no longer the habit to distress the bowels by purges, or the stomach by emetics. Here and there a few men may have a lingering predilection for depletion, and their experience may not be altogether unsatisfactory so far as certain kinds of epileptiform convulsion are concerned; or here and there a few men may still pin their faith, with some show of reason, to pur-

gatives and emetics; but these men are very few, as compared with the numbers who think that ordinary epilepsy, to say the least, must be treated in a very different manner. And why is this change? Is it that the majority had become dissatisfied with the results of a former practice? Or is it that they had come to regard epilepsy as a disease in which no good was to be expected from such measures? It is another question whether there are any forms of epileptiform convulsion which require the old mode of treatment, but this is a question which will be treated of hereafter.

Be the explanation what it may, then, a great change has come over the treatment of epilepsy, and the remedies most in vogue at present are certain preparations of zinc and copper and silver, particularly the oxide of zinc and the ammonio-sulphate of copper.

The present fancy for oxide of zinc has been caught from M. Herpin, who has devoted a substantial volume[1] to the purpose of showing that many cases of epilepsy may be cured by the vigorous and persevering use of this remedy. The doses used by M. Herpin are very large, or very soon they became so; and if they caused any inconvenience, it was only during the first few days

[1] 'Du prognostic et du traitement curatif de l'Epilepsie,' Paris, 1852.

of the treatment, when there might be a little nausea or vomiting or diarrhœa. In the case of an adult 3 grammes of the oxide are mixed with 4 grammes of powdered sugar, and divided into twenty doses, of which one is to be taken three times a day. These twenty doses serve for the first week. After this the quantity of the oxide is increased every week by the addition of 1 gramme (about 15 grains); and in this way, if the patient persevere, he will take 52 grammes in eight weeks, 132 grammes in fourteen weeks, and 327 grammes in about six months. In the case of an infant under twelve months, the quantity given in the first week is 0·25 gramme, and the addition made on each successive week is also 0·25, so that 5·25 grammes will have been taken in six weeks, 23 grammes in three months, and 68 grammes in six months. Sometimes, in consequence of the stomach being a little rebellious, it was found desirable to omit the dose taken in the morning, and once or twice it was necessary, on account of the same difficulty, to go on for longer than a week before beginning to increase the dose, but these cases were exceptional, and, when they did occur, relief was often obtained at once by giving the remedy in the form of a pill instead of in the form of a powder. And, lastly, it is a fundamental rule in this plan of treatment to persevere in the use of the remedy, and, in as short a time as possible after the cessation of the fit, to give a larger quantity than had been given previously. This is to prevent relapse. Thus, if two months had been spent in the treatment and 45 grammes of the zinc had been necessary to suppress the attack, it would be necessary to go on for another month, and, at the increased doses, to give at least 100 grammes before giving up the treatment; or, if the zinc had been given for three months, and as much as 125 grammes taken before the attack yielded, it would be necessary to go on for three months longer, and not to give up until 300 grammes had been taken.

In the work in question M. Herpin relates thirty-eight cases of epilepsy or epileptiform disease, in nearly all of which he gave the oxide of zinc in the manner which has been mentioned, and the question for us to consider is whether these cases permit us to rest content with the conclusion which has been drawn from them. The question is important, for this may be said to be the main body of the evidence in favour of zinc as a remedy in epilepsy. Of these cases, then, three are related as incomplete from the patient having been lost sight of, two as instances of spontaneous cure, seven as instances of amendment, nine as instances of failure, and *seventeen as instances of cure after treatment*, so that, setting aside the seven cases of mere amendment as not altogether conclusive, the number of cases at once falls from 38 to 17. But these seventeen are not to be taken without further reduction. Thus, one (Case 15) must be excepted as having had no zinc at all; and others (Cases 8, 14, 21, and 22) as being, to say the least, very dubious cases of epilepsy. In Cases 8 and 14 the patients were *infants,* whose ages respectively were ten months and seven months. In the first, convulsion, which had recurred repeatedly for five months, ceased immediately on taking the zinc; in the second, convulsion of three or four days' duration, recurred repeatedly during the first fortnight of the treatment, and then ceased. In Cases 21 and 22, each patient was *upwards of seventy years of age, and each patient had only one fit;* in one the person continued well for years afterwards; in the other an attack of apoplexy occurred at the expiration of three years, and the person remained hemiplegic until his death, which occurred three months afterwards, but there was no repetition of the convulsive seizure. In a word, Cases 8 and 14 may be regarded as cases of infantile convulsion rather than as cases of epilepsy in the ordinarily restricted sense of the word, and Cases 21 and 22 as cases of epileptiform convulsion depending, in all probability, upon congestion of the brain—cases, that is to say, in which it is not easy to point to the

non-recurrence of the convulsion as a proof of the
efficacy of the treatment, simply because the convulsion does not recur in such cases in the same sense
as that in which it does recur in simple epilepsy.
Indeed, as is well known, the convulsion does not
return in a great number if not in the majority of
such cases. And thus, by deducting these five
cases, the seventeen cases of epilepsy "cured under
treatment" become reduced to *twelve*. Nor is
Case 20, which is that of a lady, æt. 51, who had
one attack four or five months after the termination
of the menstrual epoch, altogether satisfactory;—
for who shall say that this convulsion was epilepsy
in the ordinary sense of the word, or that the non-
recurrence of the attack may not have been due as
much to the system having adapted itself to the
new state of things as to the medicine? Nay,
exception may even be taken to Case 6, for the patient
here was in her sixty-third year at the time of the
first attack, her conformation was apoplectic, and
the attacks themselves were evidently more of an
apoplectic than of an epileptiform character. In
this case, however, these attacks recurred at frequent
intervals for the next ten years, during which time
she did not take the zinc; and they did not recur,
except in three instances, in two of which they
were very slight, after taking the zinc. It is a
case, indeed, in which the influence of the treatment

would seem to have been very beneficial; but it can scarcely be considered as a case of ordinary epilepsy; and thus, taking these two cases as doubtful, the twelve to which the seventeen had become reduced dwindle down to *ten*—namely, Cases 7, 9, 10, 11, 12, 13, 16, 17, 18, 19. Now, in order to be able to form an opinion respecting these ten cases, and be quite satisfied that the cure was really caused by the zinc, it will be well to state what were their essential particulars.

CASE 7.—A girl, æt. 8. Four years ago she became giddy and fell, but without losing her consciousness or being convulsed. After this, such attacks occurred several times a day, with the exception of certain intervals, when they appeared to be arrested by the use of nitrate of steel. Two months before her visit to M. Herpin, she had an attack of an epileptic character, and in the week immediately preceding she had three such attacks. The oxide of zinc was given for a month, and thirteen years afterwards the report is that she had continued well.

CASE 9.—A lady, æt. 34, who had suffered from frequent attacks of vertigo during four years. For these she took the zinc. Seven years later, after having had none of her former attacks in the interval, the giddiness returned, and at last, after several partial seizures, she had a complete epileptic fit. *On this occasion powdered valerian was the remedy used.* Nine years later there had been no recurrence of the fits.

CASE 10.—A lady, æt. 31, who had suffered for ten years from occasional attacks of vertigo and petit mâl. A week after commencing the treatment these attacks had diminished; a few days later they had disappeared; ten years afterwards, or thereabouts, they had not returned.

CASE 11.—A girl, æt. 18, suffering occasionally from partial cramp in one of the hands, with a feeling like aura extending up the arm, and once or twice from an attack which seemed to be epileptic. These symptoms had been present for three or four weeks. The day after beginning the treatment she had a regular attack of epilepsy; at the end of two months, and likewise at the end of five months, she had several threatenings. Six years later she continued perfectly well in the interval.

CASE 12.—A boy, æt. 12, who had had convulsions when at the breast. Within the three months preceding the adoption of the treatment by zinc, he had had three attacks of epilepsy. Six years afterwards he had another attack, the first since the time when he had taken the zinc, and for this he was again put under the same treatment. Five years later M. Herpin reports the continued absence of fits.

CASE 13.—A boy, æt. 14½. The first attack, which was incomplete, was after having been startled by the explosion of a cannon; the second occurred a year later without any obvious cause, and the third at the end of six months from the second. At this time the zinc was prescribed. Two and a half years later the fourth attack occurred, when the zinc was resumed. Six months afterwards he had an equivocal attack of giddiness. Six years later there had been no return of either giddiness or fits.

CASE 16.—An intemperate man, æt. 21, who within a month had had two attacks of epilepsy, five partial attacks, and much giddiness. Abstinence from wine and valerian was the treatment carried out for thirty-seven days, and after this the zinc was given for nine months. During the first thirty-seven days he had five partial attacks and a good deal of giddiness; during the treatment by zinc his only annoyance was an occasional feeling of giddiness. Thirty months after this time he had a partial attack and a return of the giddiness; and two months later one complete and three partial attacks. At this time the zinc was resumed. Two days later he had three complete and three incomplete attacks, *when the zinc was abandoned, and the ammonio-sulphate of copper given in its place.* Six and a half months afterwards, feeling some giddiness, the first symptom of the kind since the last report, he was put under a course of *zinc and extract of valerian,* in equal quantities, for seventy days; and three years later there had been no symptom of relapse.

Case 17.—Another intemperate man, æt. 28, who had had three epileptic attacks within the previous four days. For these symptoms the treatment by oxide of zinc was adopted. A fortnight afterwards he had again four attacks within four days, and a month later one of a much milder character; at this time *the zinc was changed for the ammonio-sulphate of copper.* Three years later, after an interval of complete freedom since the last report, he had four attacks within four days, when *the treatment by copper was resumed.* A year later there had been no return.

Case 18.—A girl, æt. $13\frac{1}{2}$, suffering apparently from tubercle of the brain, and dying six months afterwards from general tuberculization. Every week, for six weeks before M. Herpin took charge of the case, there had been a partial attack of epilepsy, preceded by aura. After taking the zinc there was only one such attack with a little giddiness.

Case 19.—A child, æt. 9, who had had a partial attack of convulsion, without falling or losing his consciousness. The treatment by zinc was at once adopted. A month later, there having been nine such attacks in the interval, *the zinc was changed for valerian.* Eleven days later there had been six attacks, when the valerian was laid aside and *the zinc resumed.* Forty-two days later, there having been eight attacks in the interval, *the zinc was changed for the selinum palustre.* Thirty-eight days afterwards there had been only two attacks; then, after a complete interval of five years, there were two or three of the old attacks on two successive days, and after them a regular epileptic seizure. At this time the zinc was the treatment adopted; and eleven months afterwards there had been no regular seizure, and only occasional threatenings, with a few partial attacks during the earlier weeks of the treatment.

Now, on looking over these cases, it is not a little difficult to feel thoroughly satisfied as to the perfect efficacy of the oxide of zinc as a remedy for ordinary unmistakeable epilepsy. It is difficult to do this, because the cases themselves are not sufficiently marked, or in other words, the habit of convulsion is not sufficiently confirmed, to allow us to say what would be their natural course. For, assuredly, he must know little of this class of cases, who does not know that very suspicious convulsive symptoms may recur repeatedly, and subside suddenly or gradually; or that epilepsy itself may recur more than once and yet not become a habit. Even M. Herpin himself relates two cases of epilepsy coming to an end without any special treatment; and, on the other hand, he gives us the history of nine others, where the malady was really confirmed, and where, according to his own admission, the oxide of zinc was perfectly ineffectual. Nor must it be forgotten that on more than one occasion the symptoms subsided as suddenly, or almost as suddenly, under the use of valerian or selinum palustre—under the use of remedies, that is to say, which can scarcely be supposed to have any very wonderful virtues.

It would appear, moreover, that M. Herpin himself has become less confident as to the efficacy of oxide of zinc than he was in 1852, when he wrote the work from which the previous information has been taken. Thus, a more recent statement is—" que l'oxyde de zinc, ne cessant point d'être convenable pour les enfans et les viellards, échoue très souvent chez les adults." M. Delasiauve, who quotes these words,[1] tells us that the principal reason for this change of opinion was the absolute failure of an experiment in the Bicêtre, in which one of the physicians of that establishment, M. Moreau, treated eleven adult epileptics in every particular after M. Herpin's method. M. Delasiauve also tells us that M. Herpin now gives the preference to the ammonio-sulphate of copper in the treatment of adults.

Nor am I able to obtain any more satisfactory evidence in other quarters. As for myself, I may say roundly that I saw no evidence of any good results from the use of zinc in nine cases in which the metal was given after M. Herpin's plan; and that I am confirmed in this opinion, so far as epilepsy is concerned, by the result of a much more

[1] Op. cit., p. 371.

extended trial at the Westminster Hospital, by my friend and colleague, Dr. Marcet.

Of the other preparations of zinc it is not necessary to speak, for there is no evidence that they possess advantages, beyond their solubility, which do not belong to the oxide.

— Next to the oxide of zinc, the remedy at present most in favour is the ammonio-sulphate of copper. Indeed, it may even claim to rank before the oxide of zinc, for, as I have already said, the champion for zinc has become the champion for copper, as the remedy in the epilepsy of adults. It is very difficult, however, to obtain any sound evidence on the subject. Speaking of the cases recorded in his published work, M. Herpin says that, including relapses, he obtained eighteen cures in fourteen patients; but when these "cures" are fairly analysed, they do not turn out to be a whit more satisfactory than those which are said to have been brought about by the oxide of zinc. Nor do I know of anything thoroughly satisfactory in the experience of others. For myself, I ought scarcely, perhaps, to express an opinion, for I have rarely given it, and then neither in large doses nor for any length of time; but I have met with many who have taken it under advice of other physicians, and of these I have no hesitation in saying, that not a few, on being asked how they were affected by the remedy, have said, that they felt more nervous while taking it, and that no beneficial change was produced in the fits. Twelve patients have made this statement within five months.

— After the ammonio-sulphate of copper, the next rank may perhaps be given to nitrate of silver. At the same time it would seem that those who think most highly of the remedy are not disposed to risk the blackening of the skin. At the present time I have a patient under treatment whose skin is a most dismal grey from this cause, and whose fits became considerably aggravated during the time he was taking the silver; and many cases have shown that this evil may happen without any amelioration of the fit.

— Now these three remedies, zinc, copper, silver, belong to the group of diamagnetic bodies— of bodies, that is to say, which tend to arrange themselves at right angles across the magnetic meridian. They belong, indeed, to a group in which some of the companion metals are—bismuth, antimony, zinc, tin, sodium, mercury, lead, silver, copper, gold, arsenic. They belong to a group of metals, that is to say, which are all more or less sedative in their action, and this possibly may be one explanation why the result of their use in epilepsy has not been more satisfactory; for after what has been said upon the pathology of this affection, it is scarcely to be expected that a sedative remedy of any kind will be that which best suits the requirements of the case.

And if this inference be correct, is it to be expected that a remedy may be found among the magnetic bodies—among bodies of which iron, nickel, manganese, cobalt, take the highest rank? Dr. Watson says, " Of all the metallic remedies, I prefer some preparation of zinc and *iron;*" and I believe that this is the opinion of not a few in this country. I expect, moreover, that before long, iron will be tried before zinc, and not after zinc. At any rate, I may say without hesitation, that I have used iron as a fundamental element of treatment during the last seven or eight years, and that I have never seen the least evidence of harm from such a practice. On the contrary, I have often found unequivocal improvement in the general health, and as unequivocal amelioration in the fits, under a course of iron, particularly when the patient had been taking zinc or copper previously. Of manganese, nickel, and cobalt, I can only say that I have begun a series of trials, and that the medicines can be taken without inconvenience, and certainly without injury.

And if steel has done good it may be expected that quinine will be a favourite remedy. So far from this, however, quinine is not even mentioned by Dr. Watson in his chapter on epilepsy. At the same time, it has been used by more than one writer, by Rostan and Piorry among the rest, and cases are on record in which the disease is supposed to have been cured; and, for myself, I have used it almost promiscuously, and scarcely ever, if ever, without benefit. As a rule, I have given the quinine along with other remedies, about which I have to speak presently, but I have little doubt whatever that the quinine was entitled to some share of the credit.

In many cases of epilepsy, however, perhaps in all, quinine or iron, one or both, are not sufficient, and a remedy belonging to a different class puts in its claims for approval. "If," says Dr. Watson, "I were called upon to name any single drug, from which, in ordinary cases of epilepsy, I should most hope for relief, I should say it was the oil of turpentine. And I find that other physicians have come to the same conclusion. Dr. Latham, the elder, was, I believe, the first person who made known its efficacy in this disorder. Foville states that he has seen excellent effects from it. It is highly spoken of by Dr. Perceval, in the 'Dublin Hospital Reports.' It is not to be given in large doses, but in smaller ones frequently repeated; from half a drachm to a drachm every six hours."[1]

[1] Op. cit., p. 662.

Now, after what has been said upon the pathology of epilepsy and the physiology of muscular action, it is not perhaps to be wondered at that a remedy which has so positive a power of rousing the circulation as that which belongs to turpentine, in doses such as those that have been mentioned, should do good in epilepsy; but be the explanation what it may, the fact remains that turpentine is a valuable remedy in epilepsy. Of this I have had abundant evidence. Notwithstanding the evidences in its favour, however, the nauseous taste of the remedy, and the irritation which it occasionally sets up in the urinary and generative organs, have always been a serious objection to its use; and the result is, that comparatively few patients have the resolution to persevere as long as is necessary to ensure anything like a permanent benefit.

There is also another remedy which puts in its claim for approval, and this is valerian. This is a very favourite remedy, both in this country and elsewhere, and its claims, though by no means equal to those of turpentine, are in every way deserving of attention. Recommended by Aretæus and Dioscorides, and in use ever since, it was never other than a favourite remedy. Indeed, M. Herpin gives it rank next to the ammonio-sulphate of copper. Now the prominent action of valerian is that of a stimulant—an action depending upon the presence of a composite volatile oil, of which one portion is a volatile acid, capable of forming salts with bases, and known under the name of valerianic acid—and it is a natural question, after what we know of turpentine, whether this stimulating action of the drug does not show that it may be efficacious, and explain the secret of its efficacy. Be this as it may, however, as compared with turpentine, valerian can scarcely be regarded in any other light than that of a mere adjunct.

The question, then, is whether there are any remedies which possess the advantages of turpentine without the disadvantages. Is naphtha, or camphor, or ether in its various forms, or any of the stimulant gum-resins, or musk, or castor, likely to answer the end in view? Now, in an affection of so obstinate and irregular a character as epilepsy, it is no easy matter, or at any rate it is a matter requiring no little time and patience to arrive at a sound conclusion. In confirmed cases, so firmly fixed is the fatal habit, it is very difficult to make an impression; but a favourable impression may be made upon the worst cases, and I have no hesitation in saying that this impression was made by the use of the stimulant remedies in question, combined with iron or quinine, as the case may be, and associated with a generous mode of living. Under such a treatment, so far as my experience goes, the general health has improved in every case, the spirits becoming more equable and cheerful, headache disappearing, the pulse acquiring increased power, the warmth of the body being maintained with less difficulty and greater uniformity. Nor have I any hesitation in saying that an improvement in the fit was always contemporaneous with this improvement in the general health, at least in this—that the coma attending the fit became less and less profound, and the subsequent oppression or bewilderment or headache less and less distressing. I think, also, I can point to at least a score of cases in which the fits have not only been lessened in severity by being deprived of their most ominous characteristic—coma, but where the intervals between the fits have become so lengthened out, as to afford good ground for supposing that the fatal habit may be altogether broken by a continuance of the same method.

In these different trials the remedy first substituted for the turpentine was naphtha, in doses varying from half a drachm to a drachm. In the ordinary commercial form, however, this remedy proved to be scarcely less disagreeable than turpentine, and there is great difficulty in inducing patients to take it for any length of time; but this difficulty is overcome, at least in a great measure, when care is taken to procure naphtha that has been re-distilled more than once. Indeed, I may say that naphtha thus prepared may be taken for several months, without even so much as the faintest objection being raised to it. A form in which I have often given it is in combination with hop and valerian: thus—

> ℞ Naphthæ purificatæ,
> Tr. Humuli,
> Tr. Valerianæ, āā ʒss;
> Aquæ Menthæ pip., ʒss;
> Aquæ distillatæ, ʒj.
> Fiat haustus.

And in some instances, where there has been any indication for steel, I have added from five to ten grains of the ammonio-citrate of iron.

I have also had what to me was satisfactory evidence in favour of camphor. In doses of from two to six grains, either alone or in combination with quinine and iron, one or both, this remedy has rarely failed to do good. In many cases, also, it exercised, or seemed to exercise, a directly quieting influence over the generative and urinary organs —a point of no small advantage over turpentine.

Chloric ether and Hoffmann's anodyne would also seem to be adjuvants of no small value. I have often given half-drachm doses of chloric ether, either alone, or in combination with steel or quinine or naphtha. I have also found one-drachm doses of chloric ether a very effectual remedy, with or without a little warm wine and water, when it was necessary to produce some temporary stimulation. Indeed, I know of no better means of quieting the agitation which is so frequently the precursor of the attack in many of those cases which are partly epileptic and partly hysterical in their character. Of Hoffmann's anodyne I have had less experience.

Aromatic spirits of ammonia is also a valuable adjuvant, and may often take the place of chloric ether with advantage.

Of the effects of the stimulant gum-resins, and of musk and castor, I am not able to speak, not having had, as yet, the opportunity to try them, which the failure of the measures just mentioned would give, but I may appeal to their action in hysteria as an argument that they would not be useless in epilepsy.

— There are times, of course, in which a plan of treatment such as this must be suspended. If, for instance, the urine on cooling becomes thickened with lithates, not only may tonic and stimulant medicines have to be suspended, and the quantity of animal food and beer reduced, but a few grains of an alkaline carbonate, and a few drops, perhaps, of tincture of colchicum (I think I have seen much good from this addition in many cases), may be taken with advantage an hour before breakfast, for a few days in succession. Or if the bowels become obstinate, it may be necessary to recommend more fruit or salad, more walking-exercise, with enemas of cold water or brine, and so on. Or if the action of the skin flags unusually, it may be well to advise the use of a few warm baths, in addition to the ordinary practice of sponging with tepid water. In a word, any of the many minor changes which are continually happening in the system will have to be recognized and met, and not only so, but no small part of the success in treatment will always depend upon the tact and promptitude with which such changes are recognized and met.

— But what must be said of the other means which have been recommended at different times for the relief of epilepsy? What, among others (it is altogether unnecessary to notice all), must be said of strychnia, belladonna, digitalis, indigo, cotyledon umbilicus, selinum palustre, poudre de Neuchâtel, bromide of potassium, compression of the carotids, tracheotomy, cauterization of the larynx and elsewhere, chloroformization?

— *Strychnia,* as all know, was a very favourite remedy with the late Marshall Hall, but the dose was attenuated to such a degree as to render it somewhat difficult to believe that much good came from it. Dr. Hall, indeed, distinctly allows that harm is done if the dose is sufficient to produce the physiological effects of the drug. He says, "I believe it has been generally given in a dose which is stimulant (?), *and therefore injurious;*" and he will not allow more than the fiftieth part of a grain to be given three times a day. His formula is the following, the dose being ten drops:

℞ Strychniæ acetatis, gr. j;
Acidi acetici, ♏xx;
Alcoholis, ℨij;
Aquæ, ℨvj.

Such is the formula which Dr. Hall used, but after Dr. Hall's admission that the drug does harm when given in a quantity sufficient to produce a sensible action, after the admirable researches of Dr. Harley upon its *modus operandi* (p. 91), and after what has been already said in these pages upon the pathology of epilepsy and the physiology of muscular action, it is not very likely that strychnia will prove to be a valuable remedy in epilepsy.

— *Belladonna,* a remedy which was recommended by Stoerck, and used some years afterwards by MM. Debreyne and Bretonneau, has been again brought prominently into notice by no less a personage than M. Trousseau, of the Hôtel Dieu at Paris. M. Trousseau says that he has employed this remedy for twelve years, and that he has always had under treatment from eight to ten patients. He says, further, that of 150 patients so treated 20 have been cured, or, at any rate that their fits have not yet returned; and that M. Blache, who has employed it during the same period in his large private practice, has met with a like proportion of successes and failures. It is a question, however, whether 13 per cent. of successes (which may possibly, in part at least, be explained in a different way) can be regarded as sufficiently conclusive evidence in favour of the remedy, and this the more as other practitioners, among them M. Delasiauve,[1] have been less successful. Moreover, theory would seem to be against the drug, though upon such a point it is necessary to speak with much caution. For in some cases is it not possible that there may be an undue nervous sensitiveness which may be calmed by tobacco, and if so, is it not possible that up to a certain point belladonna may exercise a beneficial influence? There are some epileptics, no doubt, who may smoke with advantage if they smoke with moderation, and hence I can easily believe that there are epileptics who may, up to a certain point, be benefited by belladonna, but I cannot believe that such individuals are at all numerous. On the contrary I should rather believe that they are altogether exceptions to

[1] Op. cit., p. 370.

the rule, and that the great majority are those who cannot take with advantage, even in moderation, any kind of sedative remedy—not only belladonna, but aconite, or hyoscyamus, or opium in any of its forms.

— Another remedy upon which stress has been laid is *digitalis*, and no less a person than Dr. Williams[1] adds the weight of his authority in its favour. Dr. Williams looks upon palpitation or over-action of the heart, as a very important cause of the fit, and digitalis is one of the remedies (hydrocyanic acid is another) to which he trusts for tranquillising the circulation, though at the same time he fully allows that a permanent cure is obtained most readily by the tonic class of remedies. But, if we have read aright the phenomena of epilepsy, it is not palpitation or over-action of the heart with which we have to do when the paroxysm is imminent, and certainly there is nothing in the shape of unequivocal success resulting from the employment of digitalis which would lead us to think that this reading has been erroneous. Nor is a different conclusion to be drawn with respect to hydrocyanic acid.

— *Indigo* has also been given as a specific, particularly in Germany, and if it has not done any good it is not because it has not been given in sufficient quantity. In some cases, indeed, an ounce or more

[1] 'Med. Times and Gaz.,' 14th November, 1846.

has been given in the course of the day, and for many days in succession. But little or nothing, however, is heard of this remedy now, and the experience of many appears to be that of Dr. Pereira who says, "I have tried it in a considerable number of cases in the London Hospital, but without deriving the least benefit from it."[1]

—With regard to *cotyledon umbilicus,* there would seem to be nothing in experience, and less in the simple itself, to warrant any hope, except that which arises from the exercise of the imagination of the patient. Epilepsy requires a stronger spell than an article which might serve as an ingredient in a salad. It may, perhaps, be coerced by revolutionizing the habits, and by calling in the aid of everything which can rouse the flagging energies of the vital principle, but not by inclining towards vegetarianism. It is true that the cotyledon was tried by the late Dr. Graves, of Dublin, and that he speaks somewhat in its favour; but it failed, according to his own showing, in three out of the six cases in which he tried it; it did doubtful service in the fourth; and in the remaining two it is by no means certain that it did more good than might be expected from the hope connected with any new plan of treatment.[2]

[1] 'Mat. Med.,' 4th edit., vol. iii, p. 331.
[2] 'Dubl. Quart. Journ. of Med.,' November, 1852.

Selinum Palustre is another simple of about the same value as the cotyledon—a simple which has no place in Pereira, but which has a certain reputation in Switzerland. It is an umbelliferous plant, of which several grammes may be taken at once, and often repeated without any evident disturbance of any kind. Selinum palustre, however, is one of the four principal remedies to which M. Herpin has pinned his faith, and not only so, but it is the one to which the precedence is given in the following " ordre de mérite"—

>Selinum palustre.
>Ammonio-Sulphate of Copper.
>Oxide of Zinc.
>Valerian.

But M. Herpin gives no patent for this precedence. He says, indeed, that five of his " cures" were due to the use of the selinum palustre, but of these very five three are more nominal than real, the fits recurring in a short time, and the remaining two only claiming to be considered cures in that the fits were separated by a little wider interval than before. Indeed, this very loose way of speaking of these cases as *cures* must make us very cautious in accepting what M. Herpin says respecting the *cures* which he believes to have been brought about by the use of zinc or copper, or other remedies of unequivocal power.

The *Poudre de Neufchâtel* is another remedy which has some credit in Switzerland, and which is brought prominently before our notice by having been given in some of the cases recorded by M. Herpin. I have at present a lady under my care who took this remedy under M. Herpin's directions for several months. And what is this Poudre de Neufchâtel? It is none other than the powder of *taupe grillée,* or, in plain English, fried mole. It is, indeed, a relic of the days when, hope in other measures having failed, animal remains of a more objectionable character, fried or otherwise, were offered to the unhappy epileptic. In justice to M. Herpin, however, it must be said that he does not *believe* in this out-of-the-way remedy. He only tries it when other remedies may have failed.

Bromide of Potassium is a remedy belonging to a totally different class, and it is not suggested as of universal applicability. The suggester is no other than Sir Charles Locock, and the cases in which it is suggested are those which are called "hysterical epilepsy,"—cases, that is to say, in which there is a disposition in the fits to recur at the menstrual period, and to be accompanied with more or less excitement of an erotic character. The object is to calm this erotic excitement (the remedy being supposed to have such a power), and the dose given is from 5 to 10 grains.

"About fourteen months ago," says the baronet, "I was applied to by the parents of a lady who had had hysterical epilepsy for nine years, and had tried all the remedies that could be thought of by various medical men (myself among the number) without effect. This patient began to take the bromide of potassium last March twelvemonth, having just passed one of her menstrual periods, in which she had two attacks. She took ten grains three times a day for three months; then the same doses for a fortnight previous to each menstrual period; and for the last three or four months, she has taken them for only a week before menstruation. The result has been that she has not had an attack during the whole of the period. I have also tried the remedy in fourteen or fifteen cases, and it has only failed in one, and in that one the patient had fits not only at the times of menstruation, but also in the intervals."[1] Since this time I have given this remedy in one case, suitable so far as a very erotic disposition is concerned, but unsuitable in that the fits occurred at irregular periods, of which the longest was rarely more than a week, and the result was that fifty-one days passed without a fit. Then followed three fits on the same day, and two during the following fortnight, and there being signs of emaciation and exhaustion which were not

[1] 'Med. Times and Gaz.,' 23d May, 1853.

altogether satisfactory, the treatment was changed. It is not to be supposed, however, that a remedy whose action is very similar, if not identical, with that of iodide of potassium, can be frequently required in epilepsy, or that the power of calming erotic excitement, which belongs to the iodide as well as to the bromide, is more marked than that which belongs to camphor.

Compression of the carotids has been recommended on the supposition that a main cause of epilepsy was an afflux of blood to the head; and, among recent writers, Dr. Romberg regards it as an effectual prophylactic where there is warning and sufficient time to profit by the warning. Dr. Sieveking, also, in his recent work on epilepsy,[1] thinks that it "certainly deserves an extensive trial, . . . and that it is probable that the cephalalgia and somnoleney, which the patients so frequently complain of as distressing symptoms following the attacks, might be entirely prevented by it." As yet, however, the evidence in its favour is both scanty and inconclusive, and it might easily be frittered away by any one who is at all disposed to be sceptical.

With regard to *tracheotomy* it is less easy to come to a conclusion, and a sound conclusion is perhaps impossible, until there is a greater amount of evidence. Still, it is evident that this measure

[1] 'Epilepsy and Epileptiform Seizures;' Churchill, 1858, p. 195.

does not realize all the original hopes[1] of Dr. Marshall Hall. It does not prevent convulsion.

---

[1] The first two cases were calculated to damp the hopes of any one less sanguine and dogmatic than Dr. Hall.

The first case.—The patient in this case was a boatman, æt. 24, who had been epileptic for seven or eight years, and whose fits were frequent and severe. The operation was performed by the late Mr. Cane, of Uxbridge, during a fit of "asphyxial-coma" that had lasted nineteen hours. The relief was immediate, and for some months afterwards no fit had happened; but, unfortunately for the credit of the operation, the patient, not liking the gurgling noises and the voicelessness consequent upon breathing through the wound, *had chosen to wear the tube with its opening carefully corked-up.* This information I had from Mr. Cane himself. What the end was is not known, for soon afterwards the patient was discharged from his employment for drunkenness, and lost sight of.

The second case.—The patient in this case was a stout, thickset, muscular female, æt. 36, the daughter of an epileptic father, and herself epileptic for twenty-four years. Her complexion was ruined by the former use of nitrate of silver. The operation was performed by Mr. Anderson, of York Place, Baker Street, and the tube was worn until her death, *which happened in a fit,* about twenty months afterwards. After the operation the fits continued as before—possibly a little less frequently and severely, but decidedly of the same character. Her health and spirits are also said to have undergone some slight improvement, and she lost a numbness in the right arm which had previously distressed her, but those who knew her best doubt the existence of any appreciable change of this kind until about two or three months before her death—until, that is to say, sixteen months after the operation. The following notes of the final seizure were kindly given me by Mr. Anderson. "Eight a.m. Had been up and dressed; heard to fall heavily. A woman removed the inner tube from the trachea as she was in a fit apparently more severe than usual. She 'snorted loudly'; nails of a deeper colour. She was placed on

It does not always, perhaps usually, make the convulsion slighter. It does not prevent danger, for (as I have shown elsewhere[1]) of the few patients upon whom the operation has been performed, three have died either in the fit or in connexion with the fit, and of the three, the opening in the windpipe was free from all obstruction—at least in one. Under these circumstances, therefore, it becomes a question whether the supposed benefits of the operation are sufficient to counterbalance the associated inconveniences and dangers, even where (what rarely happens) the asphyxial symptoms are in any important degree dependent upon spasmodic closure of the glottis.

— Allowing the views which led to the adoption of tracheotomy as a remedy in epilepsy, and supposing that the disposition to spasm in the larynx, like the same disposition in hooping cough, might be overcome by *cauterizing the larynx*, Dr. Brown-Séquard was led to adopt this mode of treatment in the case of animals in which he had induced an epileptiform affection by partially dividing or otherwise injuring the spinal

---

the bed, as the woman thought she would recover as usual." The woman here referred to tells me that the patient was black in the face and violently convulsed, and that death must have taken place within ten minutes.

[1] 'Lancet,' 14th May, 1853.

marrow.[1] In animals thus mutilated it was found that a fit could easily be produced, except immediately after a fit, by pinching or pricking the skin of the face or neck; and that pinching or pricking ceased to have this effect after a longer or shorter period of laryngeal cauterization. A sponge dipped in a solution of nitrate of silver, containing 60 grains to the ounce, was applied every day or every other day, and sometimes for so long a period as three months. Dr. Brown-Séquard tells us that a third of all the animals treated in this manner were cured, and that all the rest, with the exception of two or three, were relieved; and he suggests a similar plan of treatment in epilepsy. A little later, Dr. Ebenezer Watson, of Glasgow,[2] without knowing that he had been anticipated, recommended a similar measure in epilepsy, and he relates three cases, two by himself, and one by Dr. Horace Green, of New York, in which it had actually been carried out. These cases cannot be looked upon as conclusive; but, at all events, they show, not only that the operation is practicable and unattended with any serious inconvenience, but that the fit was both slighter and less frequent during the treatment.

Dr. Brown-Séquard is also disposed to lay much

---

[1] 'Philadelphia Med. Examiner,' April, 1853.
[2] 'On the Topical Medication of the Larynx,' 8vo, London, 1854.

stress upon *cauterization in other parts,* as in the nape of the neck, and especially in the neighbourhood in which the aura originates; and he prefers the moxa or the hot iron to any milder measures. Once a fortnight, for two or three months, he would carry out this treatment, not solely, but in association with other measures. He says, moreover, that he cured of their fits two of the mutilated animals previously mentioned, by two or three applications of a hot iron to the skin of their neck. In a word, Dr. Brown-Séquard furnishes us with some additional facts in favour of counter-irritants as a means of cure in epilepsy; and not only so, but he gives a hint which may prove to be of much practical value, in pointing out the larynx, and the locality in which the aura originates, as sites in which counter-irritants *may be* especially serviceable.

Now the verdict of past experience is very much in favour of counter-irritants, and this verdict may recommend itself to the judgment, though on different grounds to those on which it is given. After what has been said, indeed, it is not easy to believe that these measures do good by withdrawing some morbid irritability from a vital organ; but it is possible that they may do good by the inflammation which they excite. It is possible that they may do this, because the fits of epilepsy are not unfrequently suspended by inflammation arising from injury inflicted during the fit or in some other way, as well as by idiopathic inflammation, and because all tremulous, convulsive, and spasmodic disorders, are suspended under similar circumstances. The occurrence of positive meningitis, for example, puts an end to the trembling of delirium tremens; the establishment of the cutaneous inflammation in small pox puts an end to the convulsions which may have attended upon the initial period of collapse; and if inflammation of the lungs is established in hooping cough, there is an end for the time to the laryngeal spasm. It is possible, therefore, and it is quite in accordance with the premises, that "counter-irritants," so called, and particularly those which excite inflammation without producing any exhausting discharge, may be beneficial in epilepsy; but I have had no actual experience in this matter.

— With regard to the treatment of the actual fit in simple epilepsy, little need be said; and, as a rule, it will only be necessary to take care that the patient does not injure himself, that the head is not allowed to hang in a dependent position, that any necklace or kerchief be unloosed. The latter precaution is of greater importance than it may seem to some, for in several cases the neck swells in the most remarkable manner from the accumulation of blood in the veins; and any ligature round the neck would be a serious impediment to the return of blood from the brain. If salt be at hand, a little may be put in the mouth; if water be within reach, a little may be sprinkled upon the face, though the advantages of such a practice are scarcely sufficient to compensate for the disadvantages and possible risks arising from wetted garments. In simple epilepsy it can scarcely ever be necessary to have recourse to chloroform, as it is in some prolonged epileptiform affections; but if it is, there is no remedy which can be more appropriate or effectual. Of this remedy, however, and of others which have been thought to be necessary when the fit is prolonged, or frequently repeated, as it is in some forms of epileptiform convulsion, it will be more convenient to speak when considering these forms of convulsion.

— In conclusion, we may say with Marshall Hall, "there is no royal road to the cure of epilepsy. The idea of a remedy for the disease is unphilosophical; and the treatment should consist in a well-advised plan, embracing every means of good, and avoiding every means of harm."[1]

[1] 'Lancet,' 30th October, 1848.

CHAPTER II.

OF TREMOR.

THE first category of convulsive disorders, in which the muscular disturbance takes the form of *tremor*, includes the tremors of delicate and aged persons, of paralysis agitans, of delirium tremens, the rigors and subsultus of fevers, and the tremblings of slow mercurial poisoning.

1. *The general history of tremor.*

The subjects of nervous trembling have a certain delicacy of constitution which cannot be overlooked; and if not women, they may be said to have a feminine habit of body and mind. It is evident, also, that they are altogether *unnerved* during the paroxysm, and that their thoughts and words are as little under the control of the will as the muscles. At this time, also, the circulation is greatly depressed, and the pulse does not recover until the paroxysm is over. Of the trembling itself nothing need be said.

Those who tremble from old age present unequivocal marks of decrepitude—the listless wish, the blanched locks, the fireless countenance, the shrunken limb, the feeble pulse, the frigid hand. Every faculty, mental and bodily, has given way under the wear and tear of life; and during the actual attack of trembling, the pulse fails, and the mind loses the small amount of power which had remained in it.

In paralysis agitans, the occasional and partial tremors of old age have become permanent and general, and in extreme cases they do not cease during sleep. If walking continues to be practicable, it is performed by stepping hastily and tremblingly upon the toes and forepart of the foot, and there is constant danger of falling from the way in which the head and body are bowed forward. And in the end, the hands, feet, and tongue fail in their proper offices, the outlets of the body are uncontrolled by the will, and the patient has to be fed and treated as a child. The paleness and chilliness, and the decided relief afforded by wine, reveal the real state of the circulation in paralysis agitans.

The trembling of delirium tremens, which is only the aggravated form of that trembling from which drunkards habitually suffer when sober, is primarily confined to the hands and limbs. It is associated with extreme fidgetiness and restlessness, and in some instances with convulsive startings. The accompanying phenomena are very marked. The hands and feet are cold, the pulse is quick and weak, the respiration is disturbed by sighs and pauses, the tongue is moist and creamy, and every movement is attended by profuse perspiration. The mind is confused, irritable, despondent, anxious, and tortured with gloomy forebodings or spectral delusions. Everything and everybody is an object of mistrust, or fear, or dread. Sleep has vanished, but the state of wakefulness is not attended by headache. In some instances there are fits of unruliness, and sometimes of fierceness, but these are easily subdued by ordinary firmness on the part of the friends and attendants. As the malady progresses, the tremors acquire the character of subsultus, the convulsive startings become more common, the coldness of the hands and feet extends to the rest of the limbs, or even to the trunk and head, the skin is more than ever drenched in perspiration, the delirium becomes low and muttering, and by quick degrees the patient sinks into a state of mortal collapse. Such is the usual course where the disease ends fatally; but in some instances these symptoms may change into, or alternate with, those belonging to meningitis, in which case the skin and tongue become dry, and, as the headache and other symptoms of inflammation make their appearance, *the tremor ceases.*

The tremors of fever and their accompaniments

are familiar to all. The rigors or shudderings at the commencement are accompanied by chilliness and paleness of the skin, blueness of the nails and *cutis anserina,* by feebleness and frequency of the pulse, by sickness and vomiting, by indescribable feelings of languor, feebleness, oppression, and by aching pains in the head, back, and limbs. The subsultus of the final stage is attended by a dusky and cool skin, a fluttering pulse, a fainting and almost silent heart, a short and sighing respiration, and by the utmost exhaustion and prostration both of body and mind.

In slow mercurial poisoning the muscles are very disobedient to the will, and all co-ordinated movements are clumsily performed. The skin is grey and dry, the pulse weak and subject to great fluctuation upon change of posture, the appetite capricious or wanting, and the whole mental and bodily strength greatly impaired. Moreover, paralysis and premature old age is the end of the unchecked disorder.

2. *The pathology of tremor.*

(a.) *The pathology as deduced from a consideration of the vascular system.*

There can be no doubt that the circulation is depressed during an attack of trembling. This is evident, as well in the paleness and chilliness of the person trembling as in the decided relief afforded by wine.

In delirium tremens, the perspiring skin, the cold hand, the quick and compressible or fluttering pulse, the treatment demanded, are all significant and unmistakeable facts. It is evident, also, that the trembling is actually connected with this state of things, for if the dry skin and excited pulse of true meningitis make their appearance, the trembling is at an end. On the other hand, an argument to the same effect is to be found in the fact that tremor is exaggerated into subsultus, or even into convulsion, as the heart and pulse fail in the course of the disorder.

Rigor, moreover, is coincident with a sense of coldness, a feeble pulse, a sunken countenance, a corrugated skin, and subsultus with a circulation faltering on the very verge of stagnation. Nor is this coincidence accidental. It is not—because the rigor disappears as the pulse and warmth return; it is not—because the subsultus may be checked for the time by the use of wine.

And in mercurial tremor an inference as to the real state of the circulation may be drawn from the general practice prevailing among the subjects of this disorder of resorting to gin and similar stimulants to make themselves steady.

— In a word, the state of the circulation in the different forms of tremor is one of under-action, and not one of over-action; and in this respect, therefore, the pathology of tremor agrees with the pathology of epilepsy, and with the physiology of muscular motion, as set forth in the premises.

(*b.*) *The pathology of tremor as deduced from a consideration of the nervous system.*

In any attack of trembling the mental faculties are all unstrung; and in the extremest forms of this trouble, as in paralysis agitans, they have altogether succumbed before the inroads of age or disease, and the patient lives only to fear and eat.

In delirium tremens the mental state is passive in every point of view. The patient is in a helpless state of fear and dread, and at every new impulse his thoughts course timidly from one object of fear to another. He lies unmanned, as it were, before some dim phantom of evil, and when a fierce delirium takes the place of the delirium tremens, and when other symptoms betoken the existence of active determination or inflammation within the skull, then the affection ceases to be delirium *tremens*, for the trembling has disappeared.

In the initial rigors of fever, the mental state is one of dejection, languor, stupor; in subsultus, it is one of wandering silliness or of drowsiness not far remote from coma.

In slow mercurial poisoning the failure of the mental power keeps pace with the failure of the bodily strength, and the condition is one of premature old age.

— In these several forms of tremor, therefore, this condition of the nervous system, as reflected in the state of the mind, is one of comparative inactivity. Nor is it easy to suppose that the condition of the brain is different from that of any other part of the nervous system, for if a due supply of blood be necessary to the exercise of the different nervous functions, as it undoubtedly is, then it follows that the medulla oblongata, the spinal cord, and every other nervous centre, as well as the brain, must be in a state of comparative inaction during the time of the trembling. With this state of circulation, indeed, it is impossible to suppose that there can be any increased supply of nervous influence to the muscles during trembling.

Nor is it an objection to this view of the matter that trembling ceases during sleep. It might seem that the trembling should continue during sleep if inactivity of the brain was one of the causes; but this is by no means a necessary conclusion. Inaction of the brain, indeed, is only one of several causes. Inaction of the circulation is another cause, perhaps a more important one, and it is possible that this cause may be remedied by the warmth of the bed. It is evident also that the brain is not called upon to make so much effort in the recumbent position as it was when it had to keep the muscles in constant action to preserve the erect position, and in this way a less amount of action on the part of the brain may be needed in the recumbent position. Nay, it may even be gratuitous to suppose that the nervous system is less active during sleep than during trembling.

3. *The treatment of tremor.*

The few remarks which have to be made under this head are altogether in harmony with what has been already said upon the treatment of epilepsy.

It is evident, in the first place, that abstinence does not form a part of this treatment. A person who trembles habitually, whether young or old, trembles more before a good meal than after it. Food, moreover, is of more importance than medicine in the treatment of ordinary delirium tremens and subsultus, and in mercurial trembling the muscular disturbance is always worse during fasting.

It is evident, also, that a glass of wine will tranquillize an ordinary attack of trembling. Wine, moreover, will steady the hand in delirium tremens, and, if the symptoms are not beyond the reach of remedies, it will calm the trembling heart and still the twitching wrist of the last stage of fever. In like manner, coffee rather than tea would seem to be a desirable remedy in all these cases.

It would seem, also, that the only remedies which are admissible in these several cases are of a stimulating and tonic character, with the exception, perhaps, of that case in which the trembling arises from slow mercurial poisoning,—with the exception, that is to say, of that case in which it may be necessary to put in practice the elegant treatment recommended by M. Melsens, and endeavour to liberate the metal from the poisoned tissues by favouring the formation of a new and soluble compound between it and iodide of potassium, which compound is afterwards eliminated from the blood by the kidneys.

— In tremor, therefore, as in epilepsy, the principal object of treatment is to avoid every cause of depression and exhaustion, to seek after every means of increasing and establishing the strength, and to trust to stimulants in any emergency.

CHAPTER III.

OF SIMPLE CONVULSION.

THE second category of convulsive disorders, or that in which *convulsion* is the distinctive feature of the muscular disturbance, may be divided (as I have already said) into two sections by the absence or presence of consciousness during the convulsion. Where the consciousness is present, the convulsion may be called *simple;* where the consciousness is absent, it is called *epileptiform. Simple convulsion,* with which we are now concerned, is that which is met with in the state called hysteria, in chorea, and in those strange affections which take an intermediate position between the two, as the dance of St. Vitus and St. John, tarantism, and other affections of the kind.

1. *The general history of simple convulsion.*

1. They who suffer from what is ordinarily called *hysteric convulsion* belong almost exclusively to the female sex, and not only so, but they possess, in an aggravated degree, the peculiar weaknesses of this

sex. They are never *strong,* and, in the majority of instances, a delicate constitution has been evidently enfeebled by disease or by some faulty habit of life.

For the most part, they are undecided, irresolute, fickle, purposeless, yielding easily and almost helplessly to every impulse either from within or from without, and scarcely ever capable of anything like sustained action. They do what they ought not to do, and they leave undone what they ought to do; and their excuse is that they cannot help it. With them *will* is little more than an empty name, and so much are they the creatures of feeling that a small matter serves to make them melt into tears or burst into laughter. The temper, also, is as little under control as the feelings, and impatience, perverseness, obstinacy, and anger are no uncommon symptoms. There is no lack of ideas; but, as a rule, these are allowed to take their own course with little check from the reason; and hence fancies and whims of all kinds in endless succession, or, what is worse, some one whim or fancy gains possession of the mind, and the reason is unable to eject it. Not unfrequently, also, there is a disposition to exaggeration and deceit which must betoken some bluntness in the moral sense if some allowance is not to be made on the ground of an imagination which cannot always stoop low enough to perceive the line which separates facts from fancies.

These mental peculiarities are all written with a certain degree of plainness upon the countenance. There is no want of brightness in the eye, no sluggishness of the pupil, no marks of "slowness" as in many epileptics. On the contrary, there is a brisk, unsteady expression which shows that the mental error is on the side, not of dulness, but of sensitiveness.

Among other evidences of an undue sensitiveness, pain and fidgetiness take a prominent place. Pain is a very common occurrence, or, at any rate, a very common complaint. It is pain in the head, pain under the left mamma, pain anywhere or everywhere in turn, seldom nowhere. Fidgetiness, also, is a common occurrence, particularly in the legs, and, in some instances, this is sufficient to make it impossible to remain in one place for any length of time. Or this want of control over the muscular system may be seen in the way a sudden noise will cause the patient to tremble or start. As a rule, also, the bodily strength is far from perfect. Sometimes, it may be, there is more strength than would appear at first sight, for any kind of exertion may be shunned from sheer idleness; but very generally there is an actual want of strength—a want which is shown both in the inability to encounter exertion and in the slowness with which the system recovers from fatigue.

The pulse is generally soft, quick, and much affected by changes of posture, becoming slower and falling, it may be, to a natural rate of frequency in the recumbent position, and resuming its former quickness on getting up. The heart is readily thrown into a state of annoying and distressing palpitation, especially by any agitation of the feelings. The circulation, indeed, is wanting in healthy vigour, and as additional evidences of this fact may be mentioned as of almost constant occurrence, paleness of the skin, coldness of the hands and feet, and a disposition to chilblains even when the weather is not very cold.

The digestive functions, moreover, are carried on in a very unsatisfactory manner. Little is eaten, and the food least liked is meat; taste is capricious, or actually depraved; digestion is tedious, and often accompanied by distressing flatulence; and obstinate constipation is a frequent trouble.

And, lastly, there are most generally unmistakeable signs of uterine derangement, more particularly excess, or suppression, or alteration of the monthly discharge.

Such are the principal features of the persons who suffer from hysteric convulsion.

2. The persons who suffer from *chorea* agree in many particulars with those who suffer from hysteric convulsion. They exhibit, often in an exaggerated

degree, the same signs of wanting will, of incapable reason, of inordinate sensitiveness. They suffer from the same timidity, the same fretfulness, the same uncertainty and irritability of disposition and temper. If there be any marked difference it is that they have less vivacity.

In many cases this want of vivacity is written upon the countenance in an expression of languor and vacancy; and in some cases this expression may be so marked that a person suffering from chorea, if seen in a moment of quiet, may almost be mistaken for an idiot. Indeed, it may be necessary in such a case to make the patient get up and move about before the true nature of his malady can be detected.

At the moment of comparative quiet the muscles in chorea are far less under control than they were in hysteria, and instead of mere fidgetiness of the legs, there is a fidgety state of every muscle in the body. The features, for instance, are distorted by frequent grimaces; the tongue is in such a hurry as to trip or stammer in its words, and if put out, it is in again before there has been any opportunity for examining it; the hand is with difficulty kept from tossing and jerking in a very inconvenient manner; and the foot will only consent to move in a starting jumping kind of gait. The muscles, also, are soft, flaccid and wasted, or at any rate they are very readily fatigued, and very slow to recover their lost power. There is, indeed, far more disturbance in the muscular system than there was in hysteria, and far less disturbance in the sensory nerves. At all events pain is by no means a prominent symptom.

The circulation is subject to considerable fluctuations, being always considerably affected by changes of posture, or by any excitement of the feelings; but any excitement is very slight and transient when compared with the opposite state of depression. The pulse, most generally, is quick and weak; the heart is readily thrown into a state of palpitation; the hands are far from a comfortable state of warmness. In many cases, also, the weakness of the circulation is further shown by paleness of the face, lips, gums, and tongue; by pastiness of the skin; by watery effusion into the subcutaneous tissue, or into the serous cavities; by murmurs in the heart and great vessels, and by other signs of anæmia; or these signs may be deepened into those of actual chlorosis. In this country, indeed, there is a connexion between rheumatism and chorea which cannot be overlooked; but this fact is not to be construed into an argument that the phenomena of fever are mixed up with those of chorea. On the contrary, chorea is essentially a feverless malady, and when it occurs in connexion with rheumatism (this will be seen presently) it is not during the occasional bouts of fever, but during the feverless overspent intervals of inaction which are habitual.

In other respects, the persons suffering from chorea resemble very closely the persons suffering from hysteria. They exhibit the same want of tone in the digestive functions. Their urine is similarly pale and copious. And if they are old enough, and of the proper sex, it will rarely happen that there is no evidence of uterine disorder.

In its ordinary form the time at which chorea is most likely to happen is between second dentition and puberty, but adults or even old persons may be the sufferers. Statistics have also shown that boys are less liable to this affection than girls.

Among the several causes, fright is assuredly the most common; indeed, chorea may be said, almost without any figure, to be only the perpetuation of that state of startling from which all suffer for a moment under such circumstances. Blows and falls on the head, and particularly irritation about the teeth, are frequently referred to as causes, and certainly there are not a few cases on record in which the symptoms of chorea have ceased on the removal of offending teeth. On the other hand, there are very few cases, except perhaps those occurring after the period of youth, in which the symptoms can be referred to any positive mischief in the central organs of the nervous system.

The history of the paroxysm.

1. The *hysteric paroxysm* is frequently ushered in by a feeling of uneasiness in some part of the abdomen, generally in the left flank,—by flatulent distension of the bowels, with disagreeable rumblings and eructations,—by copious discharge of limpid urine,—by palpitation,—by a sense of want of breath,—by an attack of actual fainting,—or by a feeling which has received the name of *globus hystericus*. This latter feeling gives the idea of a ball in the lower part of the abdomen, which after rolling about in that region for a little time, mounts first towards the stomach, and afterwards towards the throat, when it gives rise to repeated attempts at swallowing accompanied by a distressing sense of choking. Then, after screaming, or laughing, or sobbing, as the case may be, the patient begins to struggle violently and to dash herself about in the most extraordinary manner, springing bolt upright from the recumbent posture, falling back again, rolling round and round, dashing her limbs about in all directions, striking her breast, grasping and pulling at her throat as if to tear away some ligature which prevented the breath from entering, tearing her hair or garments, and sometimes striking violently at the

bystanders. She *struggles* violently, and with a degree of power that is not a little surprising, and this fact of struggling is plainly written upon the flushed cheek, the dilated nostril, and the set teeth.

All this time the patient is in a state approaching very closely to unconsciousness; but she certainly knows to some extent what she is about, though as a rule she will strenuously deny it. Indeed, a threat to drench her with water, will rarely fail to bring the paroxysm to an end. The eye, moreover, is bright and twinkling, and the pupil responds readily to light—which facts are not very compatible with complete loss of consciousness during the fit.

The circulation, for the most part, remains as it was in the intervals between the paroxysms, or if it becomes a little excited, it is far less than might be expected in such violent struggling. The breathing, on the other hand, is generally slow, embarrassed, and frequently interrupted by sobs and hiccup.

After continuing for a time, which may vary from a few minutes to two or three hours, the paroxysm generally passes off in a burst of laughter, or a flood of tears, or an abundant eructation of air, or a copious discharge of limpid urine. It is rare, however, for the patient at once to recover her small share of equanimity, and generally she will lie for some time panting and trembling, her eyes fixed and wrapt, her limbs catching and jumping, and she herself startling with a shudder at the least noise or the gentlest touch. She will lie, indeed, in a state which is the very reverse of stupor. Sometimes she may suffer for a short time from headache, from pain in the epigastrium, from a feeling of exhaustion or extreme fatigue, or from numbness or loss of motion in one or more limbs; and sometimes paroxysm may follow upon paroxysm, and at all times it is easy by any slight imprudence to bring on another paroxysm.

This is the common form of hysterical convulsion; but another form is described, and frequently met with, which is not distantly related to simple syncope. In this the patient sinks down suddenly, with slow and embarrassed breathing, but without any struggling or evident convulsion, and after lying for a moment, in which her face becomes a little flushed, and her neck a little tumid, she recovers, and after a good laugh or cry, is well again.

— When these symptoms are well marked, it is not easy to confound them with those of epilepsy. In hysteric convulsion the muscular disturbance is more that of struggling than convulsion; it is sufficiently violent, but it is quite different from the convulsion of epilepsy; it is also general : in epilepsy, on the contrary, the muscular contractions are more continued, they fix the limbs rather than dash them about, and they are more marked on one side of the body than the other. In hysteric convulsion the colour of the face is natural or only a little heightened, the features are not distorted, the eyelids are closed, the eye is bright and twinkling and its pupil is sufficiently sensitive to light, the mouth is only a little set, the lips are not covered with saliva, the neck is not twisted : in epilepsy, on the contrary, the colour of the countenance is livid, leaden, or black, the eyelid half open, the eye dull, distorted, projected, the pupil dilated and absolutely disobedient to light, the mouth dragged almost to the ear, the teeth are clenched, the lips drawn apart and covered with froth, often with bloody froth, and the whole face is twisted round so that the chin rests upon one of the shoulders. In hysteric convulsion the breathing is slow and embarrassed, frequently considerably so, but not more than this; in epilepsy it is absolutely suspended. In hysteric convulsion the paroxysm ends in a burst of laughing or sobbing, and after this the patient is left in an excitable languid state—a state which is the very opposite of anything like stupor : in epilepsy the paroxysm ends in deep coma, or rather the deep coma of the paroxysm is continued for some time after the convulsion is at an end; and after this there is for some time a stunned and stupid state of mind, with a marked disposition to sleep. In hysteric convulsion the consciousness is only partially suspended; in epilepsy it is absolutely extinct.

When, indeed, the characters of the two paroxysms are fully marked, there is little danger of confounding hysteric convulsion with epilepsy; but at the same time there is no lack of cases in which the characters of the two interblend in a very curious manner. True epileptic convulsion may indeed alternate with hysterical convulsion, and it not unfrequently happens, as the phenomena of epilepsy change for the better, that the loss of consciousness becomes less and less profound, as well as less and less prolonged, until the patient remembers something that may have happened during the paroxysm, and wakes up as soon as the convulsion is over. Indeed, this would seem to be the common mode of change for the better, in many, if not in the majority, of cases.

2. The paroxysm of *chorea* consists in certain tremulous movements, and in certain irregular and often comical or awkward shocks or convulsions. The muscles are rebellious, for they act most irregularly when they are required to carry out the behests of the will; they are also disobedient to that part of the nervous system whose office is to co-ordinate the action of several muscles in a common object, and hence such acts as handling, standing,

walking, or speaking are ill-performed, or altogether impracticable. Or the will is weak, and the organ of co-ordination only able to act in a particular direction; and hence the person so circumstanced may have to twirl about on his heels or knees, to roll side over side, to rush backwards or forwards, or to execute leaping or dancing movements, such as were exhibited in the dance of St. Vitus or St. John, in the dance which was supposed to be caused by the bite of the Tarantula, in the "Tigretier," and more recently in the "leaping ague" of certain Scotch writers, in the jumpings of certain wild religionists, and now and then in certain isolated and extraordinary cases. In ordinary cases of chorea the muscles of the face are affected first, then those of the limbs, and, lastly, those of the trunk The upper limbs are always affected before the lower limbs, and not unfrequently the upper alone are affected; the lower limbs would never seem to be affected exclusively. The movements are more marked on one side of the body, and sometimes they are confined to one side.

In the cases ordinarily met with, the muscular disturbance is partial, often confined to the eyelids or lips, and frequently not going beyond the face and neck, and one of the upper extremities. The paroxysms, moreover, are separated by wide intervals; they are not very distressing when the patient is left to himself, and when he does not attempt any unusual kind of exertion; and they cease during sleep. But, on the other hand, there are cases of a very different character—cases, happily, not very common—in which the muscular disturbance is so general and severe, that the sufferer cannot be kept in bed without being strapped down, and where no quiet can be got until the quiet is that of death. Once seen, it is not easy to forget a scene so sad as that presented by a patient thus tossing and struggling, chafed, bruised, perhaps bleeding, and never sleeping until the sleep is one from which he can only wake in another state of being.

As the disorder proceeds there is always more or less wasting in the muscles, and when the movements are confined to one side—a limitation which, according to some tables of Dr. Wicke,[1] occurred in 59 cases out of 149—the wasting was on the affected side.

As a rule, there is no stupor during the paroxysm, and even in very severe cases the patient is fully sensible of his misfortune; but in some of the more uncommon cases, there is a dreamy state of abstraction, and the mind is more or less closed to impressions from without. In all cases the will may be said to be in abeyance, and no effort is made to change or arrest the movements. As a rule, also,

---

[1] Romberg, op. cit., vol. ii, p. 51.

there is little pain, and the sense of fatigue is far less distressing than might be expected.

During the paroxysm the pulse fluctuates a good deal, and the heart often palpitates considerably, but the circulation is in no sense excited; on the contrary, the skin is rarely otherwise than pale and cool, particularly that of the hands and feet. Under ordinary circumstances the respiration appears to be but little affected, but in the severer cases it is rapid and embarrassed, and there is often a distressing sense of want of breath, which at the end of the paroxysm seeks relief in several long-drawn and sometimes sonorous inspirations.

— As in epilepsy and hysteria, the muscular disturbance may be partial as well as general. At any rate, we may perhaps mention, under the head of partial chorea, certain movements which are often considered merely as bad habits or awkward tricks, such as winking, grimacing, giggling or sneering without sufficient cause, and so on. We may also mention (for they do not seem to admit of a more relevant notice elsewhere) those uncommon cases of rhythmical contraction of the muscles of the neck by which a semi-rotatory or oscillatory movement is given to the head. Thus: the sterno-cleido-mastoid and the trapezius muscles of one side—the muscles supplied chiefly by the spinal accessory nerve—may be the seat of the disturbance, and the effect may be to rotate the head obliquely, so as to bring the ear and shoulder of that side closely together, to raise the chin into the air in the opposite direction, and to draw the head slightly backwards. These movements take place suddenly or gradually or by a succession of jerks; they continue for a few seconds, and then ceasing, they allow the head to return to its proper position until the time for the next contraction arrives. In an elderly gentleman, a clergyman, who consulted me about twelve months ago, these movements were repeated with tolerable regularity at intervals of a minute. In this case, as in such cases generally, the muscular disturbance ceased during sleep, and it might be suspended for a short time by a strong effort of the will, and by holding the head firmly between the hands; but at other times it went on in monotonous regularity without intermission. Or a somewhat similar semi-rotatory movement of the head may be caused by the rhythmical contraction of the muscles supplied by the superior cervical nerves—the splenii and obliqui capitis; or the head may go on continually bobbing or bowing forwards in consequence of contraction alternating with relaxation in the rectus capitis anticus. Muscular affections such as these are frequently accompanied with muscular contractions elsewhere, particularly in the face and in the calves of the legs; but sometimes they are the sole evidence of disorder until the patient begins to be worn out by annoyance and local pain (for the convulsed muscles are generally very painful, particularly about their insertions) and want of rest.

— The more peculiar forms of chorea—those which are distinguished by leaping, turning, or rushing backwards and forwards—are infinitely less common now than they were formerly; but still they occur in isolated cases, to the proper comprehension of which a few historical details may be of service.

The strange malady called the *Dance of St. John* appeared at Aix-la-Chapelle in the summer of 1374, and spread like wild-fire over the whole of Germany and the countries to the north-west. Hand-in-hand great multitudes of men and women went through the streets and thronged the churches, dancing and leaping, howling and screaming, until they fell down in a state of utter exhaustion. One symptom appears to have been a distressing state of flatulency, and to relieve this, when the paroxysm was over, they would entreat the bystanders to tighten their girdles, or even to leap upon them. Some had their heads filled with ecstatic visions, in which St. John was a prominent object; others were rendered frantic by certain colours and sounds.

Sometimes the dancing movements were ushered in by symptoms of an epileptiform character. For nearly two hundred years society was disorganized by persons suffering from this demoniacal epidemic, and by rogues who simulated it for sinister purposes. Dr. Hecker tells us[1] that the feast of St. John the Baptist was always held as a day of wild revelry, and that at the time when this strange malady made its appearance, the Germans were in the habit of mixing up with the Christian ceremonial an ancient Pagan usage—the kindling of the "Nodfyr." It was the custom, among other things, to leap through the flames, and to consider that a year's immunity from disease was gained by this baptism of fire. In this leaping run mad, Dr. Hecker thinks, we may find the origin of the Dance of St. John.

In 1418, close upon the heels of the Black Death, a second dancing epidemic, the *Dance of St. Vitus,* broke out at Strasburg, and, in a few days, the streets of this large city were filled with swarms of dancers, accompanied by musicians playing on bagpipes. So numerous were the sufferers, and those who pretended to suffer, that the city authorities divided them into companies, and appointed persons whose duty was to conduct them to the chapels of St. Vitus, near Zabern and

[1] Hecker's 'Epidemics of the Middle Ages;' translated by B. G. Babington, M.D., F.R.S. 8vo, London, 1844.

Rotenstein, as well as to protect and restrain them by the way. They were taken to these chapels in consequence of a legend, invented for the occasion, which represented that this St. Vitus, when suffering martyrdom under Diocletian in the year 303, had prayed for and received power to protect from the dancing mania all those who observed the day of his commemoration and fasted upon its eve. At any rate, to the shrine of St. Vitus the people went, and there priests were ready to sing masses and to perform other services fitted for the occasion. In its main characteristics the Dance of St. Vitus does not appear to have differed from the Dance of St. John.

Attention was first prominently directed to these two maladies at the times which have been mentioned, but there is good reason to believe that they were known previously.

At the beginning of the sixteenth century, a change had taken place by which these disorders were made to approximate more closely to the chorea of the present day. This is evident from the descriptions given by Paracelsus and other competent observers. At this time these maladies were characterised by a disposition to hysterical laughing or crying, and by an extravagant disposition to dance about, but without the howling and screaming and mental delusions and distressing flatulency of former days.

In some instances, also, the propensity to dance was not irresistible. Still, now and then the disorders appeared in their old form, and Dr. Hecker tells us that so late as 1623 some women were in the habit of paying a yearly visit to the chapel of St. Vitus, in the territory of Ulm, in order that a dance at the altar there might save them from dancing elsewhere until the same time next year.

Almost contemporaneously with the Dance of St. Vitus a dancing malady, called *Tarantism*, appeared at Apuleia, and thence spread with great rapidity over the rest of Italy. It was attributed to the bite of a tarantula or ground-spider common in the country; but it is far more probable that the fears as to certain supposed consequences arising from the bite—fears arising easily in the gloomy and despondent temper of the times—had more to do in causing the malady than the bite itself. Those who were bitten became dejected and stupefied; or else, becoming greatly excited, they went about laughing, singing, or dancing. In any case, they were so acutely sensitive to the influence of music of a certain kind, as to be utterly unable to restrain themselves. A kind of bacchantic furor was excited by the very first notes, and as the strain proceeded they would dance and leap and shout and scream until they fell down from sheer exhaustion. Some colours appear to have excited them, others to have calmed them. Some had a strong disposition to rush into the sea, and many were carried away by strong sensual passions into deplorable excesses. Some, again, were disturbed by the same flatulent distress as that which occurred in the Dance of St. John. In this case, music was looked upon as the only remedy, and the country everywhere resounded with the merry notes of the Tarentella. The favourite instruments were the shepherd's pipe and the Turkish drum. It was supposed that the poison of the tarantula was diffused over the system by the exercise of the dancing and expelled along with the perspiration. It was customary for numerous bands of musicians to traverse the length and breadth of the land during the summer months, and the seasons of dancing at the different places were called the woman's little carnival, "carnevaletto della donne," for it was the women, more especially, who conducted the arrangements and defrayed the expenses. Tarantism continued long after the Dance of St. Vitus had died out in Germany; indeed, it may almost be said to have been at its height in the seventeenth century.

It would seem, also, that the *Tigretier*, or dancing mania of Abyssinia, a malady occurring most frequently in the Tigré country, is not unlike the ancient dances of St. Vitus and St. John. Beginning with violent fever, this malady soon turns to a lingering sickness, in which the patient becomes reduced to the last degree of emaciation and exhaustion. This sickness may continue for months, and end in death if the proper cure be not sought after. The first cure, which is the cheapest, is one in which a priest ministers. It is a kind of water-cure, with a blessing superadded. If this fail, the aid of music is appealed to, and arrangements are made for a prolonged performance. The place chosen is generally the market-place. As the music begins the patient bestirs herself and rises upon her feet; as the performance proceeds, rapidly acquiring power, she throws herself into the maddest postures conceivable, dancing and leaping more like a deer than a human being. This she continues to do from early morning until the day is nearly spent, and the musicians altogether exhausted, when she starts off and runs until her legs refuse to carry her any further. Then a young man who has followed her fires a gun over her head, and, striking her on the back with the flat of a broad knife, asks her name, when, if cured (she had never uttered this name during her strange illness) she repeats her Christian name. After this she is re-baptized and considered convalescent. The account of this extraordinary disorder is by Mr. Nathaniel Pearce, who lived nine years in Abyssinia, who saw what he describes, and published his account about thirty years ago.[1]

A place in this strange category of disorders must also be conceded to those extravagant leapings and dancings which have been met with at different times among various sects of religious enthusiasts—the jumpers in this country and America, the convulsionaires in France, and the leapers from "leaping ague" who some time ago startled the grave kingdom of Scotland. Those affected with this latter disorder complained of pains in the head and elsewhere, and soon afterwards they began to suffer at certain periods from convulsive fits or fits of dancing. During these periods they acted as if mad, distorting their bodies in various ways, springing to a surprising height, or running with amazing velocity until they fell down exhausted. When confined in cottages, a favourite practice was to leap up and swing about among the beams supporting the roof. The effects of music do not appear to have been tested.

The time for a general visitation of maladies such as these would appear to have passed by, at least in this country, but there are still isolated cases which serve to remind us of troubles which were once more general. One of these, often

[1] 'Life and Adventures of Nathaniel Pearce.' 8vo, London, 1831.

quoted before,[1] is related by Mr. Kinder Wood, and this with two that have fallen under my own observation, shall serve as illustrations.

CASE —Mr. Kinder Wood's patient was a young married woman, who had suffered previously from headache, nausea, quick involuntary movements of the eyelids, and various contortions of the limbs and trunk. The paroxysms themselves were not always of the same kind. As the case might be, she would be violently and rapidly hurled from side to side of the chair in which she might happen to be sitting, or else thrown suddenly upon her feet, when she would jump and stamp for some time. Or, starting up, she would rush round and round the room, and tap with her hand each article of furniture that lay in her course. Or she would spring aloft many times in succession, and strike the ceiling with the palm of her hand, so that it became necessary to remove some nails and hooks which had done her an injury. Or she would dance upon one leg, with the foot of the other leg in her hand. These movements always began in the fingers, and the legs were not affected until the arms and trunk had been first seized upon. Noticing a rhythmical order in some of her movements, as if they were obedient to the memory of some tune, a drum and fife were procured, when she immediately danced up to the musicians, as closely as she could get, and continued dancing, until missing the step, she suddenly came to a stand-still. On the next occasion, a continuous roll of the drum was tried, when the dancing movements immediately came to an end, and the patient sat down. On subsequent occasions, also, the drum was had recourse to when the dancing movements showed a tendency to begin, and with the same result, so that the dancing movements, which had lasted for about a week, may

[1] 'Medico-Chir. Trans.,' vol. vii, p. 237.

fairly be said to have been stopped by the drum. Unfortunately, however, for the credit of the music, the drum and fife were found to have lost their power on two subsequent occasions on which the dancings recurred. These strange paroxysms were generally accompanied by some headache and nausea, and followed by a feeling of great weakness and exhaustion, but the patient was always able to go about her household duties in the intervals.

Case.—The patient in this case (which fell under my own notice) was a young lady between twelve and thirteen years of age, who had suffered for about three years from a choreic practice of "making faces" and bobbing her head forwards in a very curious manner. About three weeks before the date of my first visit (24th June, 1857), she suddenly began to suffer from the peculiar paroxysms which have now to be described, and a few months previously she had suffered for some weeks in a similar manner. When attacked by one of these paroxysms she would sink or rise into a sitting posture, with the legs folded under her, and then the head would be agitated by a violent alternating semi-rotatory movement, until the hair would stream out horizontally on all sides. Then followed a movement in which the whole body was thrown round and round by a succession of rapid vaults. In making these vaults the hands were placed upon the floor or bed, and the arms used as a kind of leaping-pole; and except at the instant of swinging round, when the feet and legs were thrown outwards, the half-sitting, half-kneeling posture was never abandoned. The movement of alternating semi-rotation of the head, and of circumvolution of the entire body, each lasting from one to three minutes, continued, with short intervals of rest, for about half an hour or even longer, and then she would fall back, panting and exhausted. Paroxysms such as these occurred several times a day during the first fortnight of my attendance, and then ceased suddenly. After this she rapidly improved in general health, and the choreic twitchings of the muscles of the face and the bobbings of the head became much less frequent. The improvement, however, was only temporary, and at the end of three months the paroxysms returned, though in a modified form and much less frequently. At this time, indeed, the alternating semi-rotatory movement of the head did not return, and the movement of circumvolution was varied with other movements. Thus, instead of turning, she would at times make a succession of leaps in a straight line, so that it was necessary to run in order to prevent her from falling out of bed; and now and then, after falling back exhausted at the end of the paroxysm, she would roll over and over sideways for three or four times. During these strange paroxysms there was not the least trace of stupor, and she would often complain of pain in the head, or of being excessively tired even while the muscular disturbance was at its height. In some instances during the second relapse, however, the mind was in a wrapt or entranced state, and now and then words escaped which showed that she was absorbed by some alarming dream or vision. At these times her eye had a fixed stare, and her cheeks were somewhat flushed. When the paroxysm was over she would lie for some time in an intensely nervous and excitable state, startling at the slightest noise or the gentlest touch, and now and then bobbing her head with much violence; and if the mind had been at all entranced previously, this state would continue for a short time, and then pass off with a succession of sighs. Under ordinary circumstances, however, the mind was perfectly clear, and the first moment of rest was occupied in complaining of the feeling of headache and fatigue from which she suffered. In the intervals she was nervous and excitable, but in every respect an acute, clever, accomplished, amiable girl. Her principal complaint was about a dull pain across the top of the head; an occasional complaint was about a feeling of tingling in the back and limbs. Her pulse was quick and weak, her hands and feet habitually cold, chilblains were common in only moderately cold weather, and anæmic sounds were audible in the heart and great vessels. Her appetite was very defective, and the digestion sluggish, but there were no worms nor any other evidence of derangement in the alimentary canal, beyond a slight disposition to tympanitic distension of the abdomen. Nor was there the slightest evidence of uterine derangement; indeed, the patient was in every respect a mere child.

CASE.—This case is that of a young gentleman, Mr. E—, æt. 23, who came up from the country about three years ago to consult me for what he considered to be epileptic attacks. These attacks occurred at night, and the only particulars respecting them were gleaned from his man-servant, who slept in the same room, and who said that he had been awakened more than once by hearing sounds of choking and struggling, that these sounds had ceased before he could get up, and that his master was asleep when he got to his bed-side. He had, also, other attacks, for the sake of which I now refer to the case. In the first place, he had a curious pursing up of the mouth, attended with frequent shruggings of the right shoulder and tossings out of the corresponding leg; in the next place, he had attacks of shuddering, which were so violent as to shake things out of his hand, or even to shake himself out of the chair in which he happened to be sitting; in the third place, he had what he called "a fit of turning." He had scarcely given me these particulars, when, after two or three electric-like shudders, he got up from the chair on which he was sitting, and standing upon the hearth-rug in an uncertain kind of attitude, he turned slowly round and round upon his heels for about twenty revolutions, and then sat down again. Before doing this he told me not to be surprised at what I saw, and not to attempt to stop him. He said, moreover, that the impulse to move round was not altogether irresistible, but that he felt it more easy to yield, and that he found himself less agitated afterwards if he yielded. This gentleman had gained honours at college, and there was no reason to suppose that his mental powers had deteriorated in any way. He had suffered for some time from vertigo, and occasionally from headache, but neither of these symptoms had ever been at all urgent. His pulse was 60 and weak, and during the paroxysm I have described it fell to 52 and became weaker. I noticed, also, that his respiration was somewhat impeded, and that he drew several long breaths in succession after he had sat down.

The pathology of simple convulsion.

(*a.*) *The pathology as deduced from a consideration of the phenomena belonging to the vascular system.*

1. The pulse of persons who suffer from hysteric convulsion is generally soft, quick, and much affected by changes of posture. The skin, also, is pale, and the hands and feet are subject to chilblains even when the weather is not very cold. Nor is there, as might be expected, any real excitement of the circulation during the convulsion. Indeed, the mode of breathing, which is generally slow, embarrassed, and accompanied by deep sobs and hiccup, is altogether incompatible with anything like excitement in the circulation. There is, however, in all those who suffer from hysteric convulsion a disposition to irregular distributions of blood, which distributions are sometimes inflammatory in their character. There is, indeed, a want of balance which in one sense must be regarded as another sign of a fundamental weakness in the circulation. There is, however, some reason to believe that unnecessary stress has been laid upon this disposition to inflammation in hysterical subjects; but, be this as it may, there is no reason whatever for supposing that any excitement of the circulation is connected in any way with the symptom with which we are here concerned—the convulsion.

2. As in hysteria, so in chorea, the circulation is subject to considerable fluctuations, but the habitual state is one of marked depression. The pulse, most generally, is quick and weak, and the heart readily thrown into a state of palpitation. In many cases, also, as additional evidences of a feeble circulation, the face, lips, gums, and tongue are unnaturally pale, the skin is pasty, and the serous cavities may even be waterlogged. In some instances there may be all the signs of actual chlorosis.

A disposition to rheumatism would also seem to be a common symptom in chorea. Thus, in the digest of 309 cases of chorea occurring in Guy's Hospital, Dr. Hughes says, that "out of 104 cases in which special inquiries were made respecting rheumatic and heart affections, there were only fifteen in which the patients were both free from cardiac murmur and had not suffered from a previous attack of rheumatism." Nor is it possible to get over this statement by supposing that the pain of the supposed rheumatism may have been simply neuralgic, and the cardiac murmur merely anæmic, for in eleven out of fourteen cases of deaths from chorea which are reported in this very digest, there were vegetations upon the cardiac valves. It is not to be supposed, however, that the chorea and rheumatism were actually concurrent in these cases. On the contrary, the usual statement is that the choreic patients had suffered from a previous attack of inflammation. Thus, in three cases that fell under my own notice recently, the chorea supervened in a period varying from seventeen to thirty-one days *after* an attack of slight rheumatic fever; and this was the case, also, in a case referred to by Dr. Romberg. Indeed, this connexion between chorea and rheumatism is altogether accidental, for we find this last-mentioned physician saying, that "the rheumatic predisposition noted by English medical men was rarely traceable in the cases which have presented themselves to my observation."[1]

This predisposition to rheumatism, therefore, cannot be taken as an objection to the idea, now very generally admitted, that chorea is an essentially feverless malady. Indeed, this very predisposition may be taken as an argument that the circulation in chorea is below the normal standard of activity,

[1] Op. cit., p. 64.

for, except on the rare occasions when fever is present, the circulation in rheumatism is considerably below this standard.

(*b.*) *The pathology of simple convulsion as deduced from a consideration of the phenomena belonging to the nervous system.*

1. The habitually feeble state of brain in persons subject to hysteric convulsion is shown in a variety of ways—indecision, irresoluteness, fickleness, pliability, over-sensitiveness, fidgetiness, and so on. And in the fit, the will is altogether in abeyance, and the mental state is one approaching very closely to unconsciousness. Nor is it easy to suppose that any part of the nervous system can be in a more excited state; for, as in the case of epilepsy and the different forms of tremor, the state of the circulation at the time of the convulsion is incompatible with the existence of anything like high functional activity in any organ, nervous or other.

In a word, there is nothing in the history of hysteric convulsion or its antecedents which does not harmonize with the history of epilepsy and tremor, and their antecedents; and there is no necessity to suppose that the uterus has anything to do with the phenomena of the so-called hysteric convulsion beyond this—that many common and important causes of weakness and exhaustion refer more or less directly to this organ. Nor is the hypothesis of "morbid irritability" more necessary to explain the phenomena of hysteric convulsion than it was to explain the phenomena of epileptic convulsion.

2. The persons suffering from chorea present the same evidences of mental feebleness as those which were met with in hysteria—the same vacillation, irrationality, inordinate sensitiveness, timidity, fretfulness, irritability. It is to be supposed, also, that this mental state is a fair representation of the state of all the nervous centres, for the circulation is manifestly unequal to maintain the action of these centres at the normal pitch.

Nor is any evidence of a contrary character in the background, if that evidence be fairly examined. In the fourteen cases of deaths from chorea contained in Dr. Hughes' digest (which cases may be said to constitute more unexceptional evidence on the subject than any other on record) the brain was quite healthy in four, and only congested in three others, so that we may conclude that there was nothing the matter with the brain in half of the whole number of cases. And of the remaining seven cases the particulars are as follows: serous effusion beneath the arachnoid and into the ventricles, slight effusion of blood beneath the right cerebral hemisphere, softened brain;—arachnoid opaque, brain dark and soft;—pia mater watery, cineritious matter red, soft, and partially adherent;— brain soft and vascular, much fluid in ventricles;— arachnoid opaque in parts, cerebrum vascular, left thalamus rather soft;—dura mater adherent very firmly to calvarium, and more opaque than natural, cerebral vessels turgid;—blood effused into arachnoid, fornix and edge of third ventricle soft, red, and tumid, brain softened. In the same fourteen cases the spinal column was not opened in six. Of the remaining eight the cord and its membranes were quite healthy in three, and only a little congested in one, so that there was nothing the matter with the spinal cord or its membranes in half the number examined. Of the remaining four the particulars are these: soft adhesions of the arachnoid, grey matter dark;—vessels rather large and numerous, serous surfaces opaque, old adhesions of the membranes, especially posteriorly;— medulla slightly softened, rachidian fluid opaque, yellow, and densely coagulable by heat;—softening of the cord opposite the fourth and fifth dorsal vertebræ. In half the number of cases, therefore, there are signs which show more or less clearly the presence of inflammatory changes during life, but it is not possible to assume that these changes have any essential connexion with the chorea, and this for no other reason than that they were wanting in the other half of these very cases. It may be, indeed, that the inflammation preceded the chorea, and left the cord damaged and to that extent weakened, and this opinion would not seem to be improbable where the signs of mischief were evidently of no recent date; or it may be that the inflammation had been a consequence rather than a cause of the chorea,—the cord, like the muscles, breaking up, as it were, from sheer fatigue. Or, possibly, the appearances as of inflammation, if they had been more carefully noted, might have been explained without the hypothesis of inflammation at all. At all events, this hypothesis would seem to gain but scant support from the history of the symptoms during life.

In the present state of physiology it is scarcely possible to speculate successfully upon the causes of those strange co-ordinated movements, such as turning or rolling, which in one sense come within the category of chorea. It is found[1] that turning or rolling *towards the injured side* is caused by puncturing the anterior extremity of the thalamus opticus (Schiff), the crus cerebri (Majendie), the tubercula quadrigemina (Flourens), the pons varolii, the posterior part of the processus cerebelli ad pontem and the auditory nerve (Brown-Séquard), the medulla oblongata at the point where the facial

[1] Brown-Séquard, op. cit., p. 19.

nerve is inserted (Brown-Séquard and M. Magron), the medulla oblongata on the outside of the anterior pyramids (Majendie), and a greater part of the posterior surface of the medulla oblongata (Brown-Séquard). It is found, also, that turning or rolling *from the injured side* is caused by puncturing the posterior extremity of the thalamus opticus (Schiff), the crura cerebri (Lafargue), the anterior part of the processus cerebelli ad pontem, and a small part of the medulla oblongata before the nib of the calamus scriptorius and behind the corpora olivaria (Brown-Séquard and M. Magron). The results are strange, but for the most part they are constant. It is enough to make a puncture and the animal turns, or (what is an exaggeration of the same thing) rolls. As Dr. Brown-Séquard has pointed out, the muscles on one side of the body are more contracted than the muscles of the other side under these circumstances, and the rotation is partly due, in all probability, as this physiologist would have us believe, to the fact that the animal cannot move in a straight line because the muscles of the two sides contract with different degrees of force.

Now, there is no time for inflammation to be set up in these experiments, and after what has been said previously, it is difficult to suppose that the knife has acted by irritating the mutilated organ, in the sense of exciting it to a higher degree of action. On the contrary, the whole tenour of the previous argument has been to show that a mechanical agent produced contraction by a process which is more akin to exhaustion than stimulation; and there appears to be nothing in the case under consideration which need militate against this conclusion. Nor is a different conclusion required where the choreic movements are connected with "irritation" in the gums, or alimentary canal, or uterus, or other organ, for here also there is the same necessity for regarding the *modus operandi* of the morbid process as exhaustive in its character, not stimulative.

There are many points in the pathology of chorea and the allied affections upon which it does not do to dogmatize in any manner, but the facts so far as they may be apprehended are in harmony with the previous considerations respecting hysteric convulsion, and tremor, and epilepsy; and the pathology throughout, so far as we have yet gone, is in keeping with the physiological considerations respecting muscular motion. It is still muscle contracting because "nervous influence" is withheld, and not because "nervous influence" has been imparted.

The treatment.

1. In the treatment of hysteric convulsion it is manifestly of primary importance to correct, as far as may be, those erroneous habits which have led to the disorder, and because this is no easy task, the results of treatment are by no means so certain and satisfactory as might be expected. Exercise, early hours, useful occupations, other reading besides novels, and strict temperance in all matters relating to the emotions and appetites—a rule of life, indeed, rigorously in accordance with the dictates of common-sense—all this must be insisted on and realized before much good can be done. In matters of eating and drinking there seem to be no sound reasons for supposing that a different rule is necessary to that which is ordinarily observed in this country, but if there be, it is not a rule requiring less wine and stimulants than usual. Indeed, there are many cases, especially those in which the strength is continually kept down by profuse menstruation or leucorrhœa, in which stimulants, in no stinted quantities, must be regarded as necessaries of life.

It may be questioned, moreover, whether the practice of giving purgatives is so beneficial as it is supposed to be by some. Aperients may be very necessary, and active purges may now and then do no great amount of harm, but neither aperients nor active purges are in much request if care be taken to prevent the diet from being too unstimulating and the habits from being too sedentary. At any rate, according to my own experience, the bowels under these circumstances will act well enough without any aid from aperients or purges; the stomach would even seem to do its work all the better for being allowed to do it in peace; and hysteric convulsion would seem to be a less frequent occurrence.

It may also be questioned whether the use of the shower-bath is called for in the majority of cases. If there be no objection to it on the part of the patient, and if reaction be established at once, it may do good, but where the patient shrinks from the shock and is slow to recover her warmth, the benefit would seem to be very problematical. I think, indeed, that I have seen several cases in which positive good has resulted from its discontinuance.

It is no doubt a matter of extremest moment to correct any uterine derangement, and in order to do this, as it seems to me, we cannot be too chary in having recourse to measures which may serve to give an undue prominence to uterine matters in the imagination of the patient. Common measures used in the common old-fashioned way, particularly

12 §

if the diet be not too unstimulating, will rarely fail to set matters right.

The other symptoms are such as to indicate the necessity of tonics for the most part, especially iron, and few are now deterred from the use of these remedies by any scruples about plethora and irritation. If pain be a prominent symptom, anodynes may be required, as opium in one or other of its forms, henbane, &c., and these remedies will be found to agree much better than they do in epilepsy; but as a rule, perhaps, the pain will be best quietened by the remedies which are had recourse to for removing the spasmodic symptoms—ether, ammonia, valerian, assafœtida, or, it may be, wine. Indeed, the principles of treatment are in no essential particular different from those which have been advocated when speaking of epilepsy, except that more may depend upon a radical reformation of the habits of the patient and less upon the use of medicine.

In the convulsion itself little need be done beyond loosening the stays and sprinkling cold water in the face; but if more is required, as when fit succeeds upon fit in spite of all ordinary measures, there is nothing better than the plan recommended by Dr. Copland, which is to throw up an enema, consisting of half an ounce or an ounce of turpentine in a little gruel, or milk, or broth.

2. " When," says Dr. Watson, in his chapter on chorea, " a vast number of different drugs are recommended as specifics in any given disease, we may sometimes infer from that very circumstance that the disease is difficult of cure, and generally untractable under all plans of management. But there is another class of diseases which a variety of drugs are supposed capable of curing—those which tend to terminate in health. I believe, also, that many of the boasted specifics have been quite innocent of any share in the recovery of the patients to whom they were administered : at the same time, I am quite certain that treatment has a great influence over the disease."

Where there is a fixed pain in the head, Dr. Watson recommends the local abstraction of blood, but, with this exception, he considers that " bloodletting is neither useful nor even satisfactory." Indeed, he allows that there is " a deficiency rather than a redundancy of red blood in the system." He says further that, setting aside this complication with headache, most of the cases of chorea may be dealt with successfully if we have at our command purgative medicines, the cold shower-bath, preparations of iron and arsenic, and the oil of turpentine. " The instrument," as Dr. Watson says in another place, " is not broken anywhere, but slackened,

[1] Op. cit., vol. i, p. 675.

jangling, and out of tune; and (to pursue the metaphor) we often can restore its harmony by bracing it up again."

It may be a question, however, whether leeches are required even in exceptional cases, whether purgatives given by the mouth do not derange the stomach to a degree for which there is no compensating advantage, and whether the shower-bath is altogether innocuous; for an opposite plan of treatment would seem to answer the end as well,—if, as Dr. Watson believes, " there are *cures* in the disease as well as recoveries." At least, I have been in the habit of placing most confidence in stimulants for some time back, and apparently this confidence has not been misplaced. The following case, the last in my case-book, and the counterpart in essential particulars of three occurring within twelve months, may be taken as an example:

CASE.—S. T—, æt. 17, was admitted under my care into Burdett Ward, Westminster Hospital, on the 6th of January, 1858.

About two months previously he began to complain of pain and weakness in the ankles, and for these symptoms he went to the Orthopædic Hospital, and was recommended to wear strong boots with irons up the legs. A few days later his speech became hesitating, and the limbs were jerked about in a ludicrous and awkward manner. Ten days ago these latter symptoms were considerably aggravated, and at the advice of a physician of eminence he was put under a treatment consisting of daily purges of croton oil, with cod-liver oil and digitalis. It appears, further, that he had suffered for three or four years from frequent headache and epistaxis.

On admission, the expression of the countenance was so vacant as to suggest the idea of idiocy—an idea not a little confirmed by the fact that the saliva was allowed to dribble from his mouth without any effort to wipe it away. His grimaces were extraordinary, and the tossings of his head and limbs and body were such as to make it difficult for him to sit in a chair while the bed was being got ready. If spoken to, his apprehension appeared to be very slow, and his speech was so "thick" as to be unintelligible. The tongue could not be held out for a single instant. The hands and feet were very cold; the pulse was 72, weak; the heart's action normal; the appetite good. The treatment recommended was the following draught:

℞ Naphthæ purificatæ, ʒj;
    Ferri ammonio-citr., gr. xv;
    Aquæ menthæ pip., ʒj;

every four hours, a turpentine enema every night, with wine and full diet.

January 7th.—The sleep has been sound and refreshing throughout the night. The enema operated well. Pulse 88, stronger. Speech more intelligible. Agitation of the arms and head less marked.

8th.—Another good night's rest. The tongue can be kept out without much difficulty. The arm can be held out with comparatively little jerking. Pulse 88, stronger. Enema brought away more fæces of a dirty mud colour. None of the evacuations following the enema have been copious, and the patient says that the effect of the enema is to make him warm for two or three hours. On enquiring as to the effects of the purgatives given to him before he came into the hospital, he said that they had made him feel sick, and that they had increased the agitation and taken away his appetite.

13th.—This afternoon he is sitting up in a chair, and on being told to get up and walk along the ward, he did so with very little assistance. The tongue is now protruded naturally, and there is scarcely anything wrong with his speech. The enema to be discontinued.

19th.—The choreic symptoms have altogether disappeared, the speech is quite distinct and clear, the countenance has lost altogether the vacant expression it had upon his admission. Convalescent. The naphtha and steel draught to be changed for another containing quinine and steel.

I have adopted a similar treatment to this in several cases, with similar results, though not always with such speedy success. I also gave naphtha along with tincture of valerian and hop in the remarkable case in which the principal symptoms were alternating semi-rotation of the head and circumvolution, and apparently with the most marked benefit in the first instance, for the symptoms suddenly came to an end in a few days. I had, however, less reason to be satisfied with it in the relapse, when the symptoms were less purely choreic and more hysterical in their character.

Of arsenic I have had little experience, and that simply because the symptoms have yielded to the treatment described before I had time to become doubtful as to its efficacy.

In all cases, of course, it is necessary to look for

and remove all sources of "irritation," such as carious teeth; and, in cases of partial chorea, the aid of the surgeon may be necessary, not only to remove carious teeth, but to divide offending muscles.

In many cases, generous living, moderate exercise, abundance of sleep, and a merely nominal treatment, have served to bring about a "cure," upon leaving off the cold shower-bath and ceasing to "regulate the secretions" by a too assiduous devotion to purgative remedies.

CHAPTER IV.

OF EPILEPTIFORM CONVULSION.

Epileptiform convulsion, as we have already said, agrees with simple epilepsy and differs from simple convulsion, in that it is attended with loss of consciousness. It may occur in connexion with certain diseases of the brain—chronic softening, chronic meningitis, tumour, induration, hypertrophy, atrophy, congestion, apoplexy, inflammation—with fever, with certain retained excretions, with "irritation" in the gums and elsewhere, and with the moribund state; and a clear view respecting it is only to be obtained by considering it in these several connexions.

The history of epileptiform convulsion.

1. The persons in whom epileptiform convulsion is a sign of *chronic softening of the brain* are never young. If not advanced in years they are prematurely old. Under all circumstances there is unquestionable, often very marked, impairment of the intellectual faculties, and, in extreme cases, the mind may be a complete wreck. Fire and energy

have died out, and dulness and drowsiness point to the coming coma of which they are the forecast shadows.

Paralysis, generally of a hemiplegic character, is the constant accompaniment of this mental blight—paralysis which, as a rule, differs from the paralysis of hæmorrhage in being more slowly developed, as well as in being less complete and less uniformly unchanging. At one time or another, also, and generally, but not always, on the paralysed side, there is more or less permanent spasm; but this symptom is not always present, and, most assuredly, it is not that diagnostic sign of softening which it was once supposed to be. Trembling and shuddering are also occasional symptoms.

Pains in the head are rarely absent, and pains in the limbs and paralysed muscles are common troubles. In the head, the pain is rarely more than a dull aching diffused over a considerable portion of the scalp, and sometimes it does not amount to more than a sensation of weight. It is often spoken of as rheumatic, and so also are the pains in the limbs. In other respects the nerves of sensation do not appear to be much affected. There is often an arcus senilis in the eye, but vision is not often seriously damaged, and hearing and feeling are less affected than might be expected from the extent of the paralysis.

Of the other appearances which may be noticed during life, the principal are those which indicate a feeble circulation—extremities habitually cold, cord-like arteries from atheromatous changes in their coats, a weak and probably fatty heart, and so on.

In this condition the brain is pallid, whiter than it ought to be, deficient in red spots, and in parts softer than natural, sometimes even diffluent. These parts are more commonly met with in the medullary or least vascular portions of the cerebral tissue, and their locality is not at all determined. Examined microscopically, the softened substance is found to consist of broken-down brain tissue, with a greater or less number of cells containing oil, and sometimes with few or many blood-corpuscles (for hæmorrhage is a common consequence of softening), *but without any of the products of inflammation,* such as exudation-corpuscles and pus-corpuscles. The colour of the softened portions will be pale or red in various shades, according to the quantities of blood mixed in them. Atheromatous and calcareous deposits are also common in the vessels of the brain.

— The epileptiform convulsion which occurs in chronic softening of the brain is usually less violent than that of simple epilepsy, but not always. Consciousness is completely lost, and the subsequent stupor passes off very slowly. Recovery, indeed, is imperfect as well as tardy, and the mental confusion or paralysis which existed before the fit is generally aggravated by the fit. In a word, the effects of the storm do not pass off so speedily and (in a sense) so completely as they do in epilepsy, though it often happens that the symptoms of suffocation and cerebral congestion during the fit itself are less urgent.

2. *Chronic meningitis* is generally met with in children or in young persons, and not in persons past middle age, as is the case with chronic softening of the brain. It is usually accompanied by evidences of a scrofulous habit, and not unfrequently it would appear to have originated in some local mischief, such as disease in the bones of the ear.

As in chronic softening of the brain the most prominent symptom is progressive impairment of the mental faculties, but in chronic meningitis this impairment would seem to be attended by peevishness, impatience, fidgetiness, and a disposition to delirium, rather than by dulness. At one time or another mental wandering in the evening or at night is a common symptom, and not unfrequently this wandering may be exaggerated into actual insanity. It would seem, also, that convulsion occurs more commonly than it did in chronic softening of the brain, and that spasm and paralysis occur less frequently. At an early stage of the disease there will often be twitchings or contortions in the features, or squinting, or some tripping of the tongue, and at an advanced stage there may be a palsied limb,—this being, in all probability, the extent of the mischief in this direction. It is no unusual thing to find the flexor muscles of the paralysed limb permanently contracted, and the whole of these muscles unduly sensitive to percussion; but spasm, either permanent or transitory, is not a prominent phenomenon. Headache is rarely absent, and the pain is very much of the same character as it was in chronic softening—dull, and not confined to any one spot in particular. Vertigo is a frequent phenomenon.

The pulse, for the most part, is quick, weak, and greatly affected by changes of posture, as indeed is to be expected from the state of weakness and exhaustion which is invariably present. In the evening faint hectic reaction is a not uncommon condition, when the cheeks become flushed, the eyes brilliant, and the aching head hotter than it was before; and this faint hectic reaction is one of the points in which chronic meningitis differs from chronic softening. Moreover, nausea, vomiting, and constipation are not uncommon symptoms.

— The epileptiform convulsion which occurs in chronic meningitis may be general and accompanied with complete loss of consciousness, but in many instances it is confined to a part of the body, and some degree of consciousness is retained throughout the paroxysm. In a case recently under my care, the convulsion never went beyond the most extraordinary agitation of one arm, and though utterly unnerved and wholly unable to control herself, the patient remembered everything that had happened during the fit. In a case like this, or in any case where the state of coma is absent or incomplete, there is no consecutive stupor; and it would always seem to be a marked difference between the convulsion arising from chronic meningitis and the convulsion arising from chronic softening, that the consecutive stupor is not a marked phenomenon in the former instance.

Chronic hydrocephalus is closely akin to chronic meningitis, and, like it, is a passive rather than an active affection. Its affinities, indeed, connect it with atrophy, and not with any inflammatory changes, for the brain is, for the most part, wasted, the membranes unchanged or only slightly opalescent, and the effused fluid is simple serum highly diluted with water. Or if there are evidences of structural change in the membranes or elsewhere, the microscope shows that the change is of a tuberculous character. If the affection be congenital and life prolonged, the child is in all probability blind, deaf, dull, idiotic perhaps, and paralysed; and it would seem to be a rule that the frequency of convulsion is directly related to the degree of the marasmus.

3. *Tumour of the brain* may be of several different kinds—tubercle, cancer, &c., or it may be hydatid or aneurismal in its character. Tubercle, which is by far the commonest kind of tumour, is generally met with in children and young persons, and where it is met with, it is rarely a solitary manifestation of the scrofulous habit. Cancer, which ranks next to tubercle in order of frequency, is oftener met with in persons advancing or advanced in life, and as was the case with tubercle, the deposit in the brain is rarely the only evidence of the constitutional disease. The other kinds of tumour are comparatively uncommon, and when they do occur their character is only to be guessed at inferentially. Thus, aneurism may be suspected if the vessels elsewhere furnish evidence of similar enlargement.

The symptoms of tumour vary greatly, and in many cases, where the development has been gradual, the very symptoms which are regarded as most characteristic may be wanting.

In the majority of cases the intelligence does not suffer in any marked degree, and when it is otherwise it would seem to be owing in great measure to the presence of chronic meningitis. In many cases the several major faculties of the mind —feeling, judgment, fancy—are comparatively unscathed, and a slight tinge of melancholy or irritability may be the only evidence of the existing mischief. Convulsion, on the contrary, is a common phenomenon—a phenomenon as common as in chronic meningitis, and much more common than in chronic softening. Convulsion, moreover, is much more common than spasm or paralysis,—indeed, this comparative want of spasmodic or paralytic disorder is one of the evidences of tumour. Convulsion is most common, as it would seem, when the cerebellum is affected. Headache is another prominent phenomenon, and the pain is of a particular character. It is not dull diffused aching, as in chronic softening or meningitis; it is severe and confined to one spot, with frequent pangs of a violent and almost intolerable character. These pangs are readily brought on by any effort, mental or corporeal, by emotional excitement, by a glare of light or anything of the kind. Vertigo is another common phenomenon. In some cases, also, the optic nerve, or some other nerve, special or general, may be paralysed by the pressure of the tumour.

The person suffering from tumour of the brain is generally weak and exhausted from the pain, or want of sleep, or mental depression, one or all. The pulse is quick, weak, and irritable, fluctuating considerably in the twenty-four hours, and occasionally exhibiting a slight hectic quickening in the evening, particularly when the tumour has given rise to any symptoms of chronic meningitis. Want of appetite, nausea, vomiting, constipation, may also accompany this hectic quickening, but all these symptoms would seem to be more connected with collateral conditions than with the tumour itself.

It is very difficult, if not impossible, to determine with any exactness the position of the tumour. Pain, or amaurosis, or any other affection of one of the nerves of special sensation, is most commonly upon the same side as the tumour, and the palsied or rigid condition of the limbs on the opposite side, but this rule has frequent exceptions. Generally the pain is referred to the neighbourhood of the tumour, but the pain connected with a tumour in the cerebellum has been seated in the forehead. "Upon analysing a considerable number of cases," says Dr. Reynolds, in his very admirable work upon the 'Diagnosis of Diseases of the Brain,' "I find that convulsions are most frequent in tumours of the cerebellum, and that they diminish in frequency as the seat of lesion advances forwards—that is, through the posterior and middle to the anterior lobes of the cerebrum. Amaurosis, on the other hand, is most common in tumour of the anterior cerebral lobes; and it becomes relatively less frequent as the seat of the tumour retrogrades. The same is true, to a certain extent, with regard to impaired intelligence and articulation." If the tumour be at the base of the brain, there is a greater probability that the nerves of special sense will be affected. Dr. Romberg says that the pain is increased by forced *ex*piration when the tumour affects the upper surface of the brain, and by forced *in*spiration when it affects the under surface. And many think that tumours in the meninges are especially characterised by pain and convulsion, and tumours in the substance of the brain by greater disturbance of the mental faculties, by more marked paralysis in the special or general system of nerves, but, as Dr. Reynolds says, " the data upon which this opinion is founded are unsatisfactory." Nor does vertigo or vertiginous movement point to any one particular part of the brain, as indeed we may expect from the fact that turning will result from so very many different injuries of the brain.

— Epileptiform convulsion is a common occurrence in tumour of the brain, particularly in the advanced stages of the disease. In the few days preceding death, indeed, convulsion may succeed to convulsion, with scarcely any interval. The paroxysm may be violent and general, as in ordinary epilepsy, or it may be irregular and confined to the head and upper part of the body. In the general attacks the loss of consciousness is complete, and the after-stupor profound; but in the slighter and more partial forms, the consciousness is often partially retained, much to the distress of the patient, who greatly dreads those attacks in which there is consciousness of the sad struggle of which he is the subject. It is, indeed, the rule for the after-stupor to be much less marked in tumour than in simple epilepsy and chronic softening, except perhaps for a day or two preceding death, when the patient is lying, in all probability, in a moribund state. It is a rule, indeed, for the fit to be followed by depression and increased pain in the head rather than by actual stupor.

— Under the head of tumour, perhaps, it may be convenient to allude to those cases in which epileptiform convulsion is caused by the depression of a portion of the skull upon the brain. In cases of this kind the patient is left in a comatose state, which may easily be mistaken for apoplexy by a person who is unacquainted with the history, or who does not examine the head carefully; and if convulsion happens shortly after the injury the circumstances are in every respect similar to those which attend upon the convulsion which may happen in apoplexy, of which circumstances more will be said presently. If convulsion happens at a later period after the injury, the patient may have recovered more or less completely from the state of coma and paralysis, and the probability is, that some diseased state, inflammatory or non-inflammatory, acute or chronic, has been set up in the brain, and that the convulsion is symptomatic of this state.

4. Workers in lead, or those who have been drinking water that has been poisoned by leaden water-pipes or cisterns, and a few who have taken lead for medicinal purposes, are sooner or later affected very injuriously. A general state of cachæmia is induced, the muscles waste and lose their irritability, and at the same time they become subject to tremor, spasm, convulsion, and, last of all, to paralysis. In this change the extensors are affected more than the flexors. This state of bodily decay is attended by marked failure of the intellectual faculties, and when the brain is examined after death, it is found to be harder, darker in colour, drier, more bloodless, andcontaining an appreciable quantity of sulphate of lead. A similar state of *induration of the brain,* without the presence of the lead, has also been met with in cases of epilepsy where there was no reason to suspect the presence

of lead-poisoning, and some authors have gone so far as to say that the brain is always more or less indurated in this disease.

The convulsion, which is a common occurrence in this state, has nothing to distinguish it from ordinary epilepsy, or if there is anything it is only in its greater violence.

— These cases of induration of the brain are often spoken of as cases of hypertrophy of the brain. According to this view it is supposed that the brain has become harder because it had no room to expand, and the flattened state of the convolutions, a not unfrequent appearance, is pointed to as an argument in favour of this view; but it is more easy to believe that the proper tissue, instead of being hypertrophied, is actually atrophied, and (as Dr. Bucknill has pointed out in certain cases of insanity[1]) that the enlargement of the brain may be owing to the growth of structures of an inferior quality. In children, however, there are no doubt cases of true hypertrophy of brain, where the bones have yielded, and the head has acquired an appearance which is very similar to hydrocephalus; but such cases are rare, and the patients so suffering do not appear to have had any other inconvenience

---

[1] A paper on the "Pathology of Insanity" in 'British and Foreign Review,' January, 1855.

beyond the deformity. Two cases of the kind are quoted by Dr. Watson.

5. *Atrophy of the brain* may be a congenital condition, or it may be brought on by pressure, as in the case of chronic hydrocephalus or tumour, by the obliteration of arterial trunks, as in those cases of arterial plugging to which attention was first directed by Dr. Kirkes, or by other means of a more recondite character. Where it is congenital the wasting, or rather the want of development, is usually more marked in one hemisphere than the other, and in this case the opposite side of the body is shrivelled and some of its muscles contracted. In this case, also, the patient is generally both idiotic and epileptic. Of the other cases of atrophy our knowledge is not sufficiently positive to enable us to speak with any degree of precision.

6. *Congestion of the brain* is an affection which belongs to declining years rather than to early life. A person so suffering is less "bright" than he was, confused instead of clear in his ideas, wanting in the power of attention, drowsy, and these symptoms are aggravated by stooping or lying down. He suffers, also, from vertigo, dulness of hearing, dimness of sight, weight and aching in the head, lassitude, and other symptoms of the same kind; but not from any kind of delirious disturbance. His head and face are injected and dusky, his

features torpid, his jugulars full, his pulse and respiration slow and laboured, his hands and feet habitually colder than his head, his bowels in all probability constipated. These symptoms may fluctuate a good deal, and at times pass off altogether; but, sooner or later, severer symptoms are brought on by some unusual bodily effort, as in straining or stooping, or by some strong mental or emotional excitement. These severer symptoms are similar to those which belong to cerebral hæmorrhage; in other words, consciousness is suddenly lost, and the body falls paralysed and senseless. These symptoms, indeed, only differ from those of cerebral hæmorrhage in that the consciousness partially returns, and the paralysis and numbness partially pass off after the lapse of a few minutes. It is the rule for the paralysis to be general—that is, not confined to one side, and for none of the muscles to be rigid. It is the rule, also, for these symptoms to pass off in a short time without leaving any of the limited and permanent paralysis which is consequent upon hæmorrhage or softening. In a short time, indeed, and after a little increased dulness, headache, and muscular feebleness, the patient returns to his former state. Such is the usual course of the severer symptoms belonging to congestion, but it is not the constant course. In some instances, indeed, these symptoms may have an epileptiform instead of an apoplectic character, and the convulsion may be very violent. According to Durand Fardel this attack is not ushered in by a cry, but the cry is no distinctive feature of ordinary epilepsy, as he supposed, and a cry was certainly present in several instances of epileptiform convulsion arising from cerebral congestion in a patient (æt. 53, and whose first attack occurred twelve months before,) recently under my care. It is also questionable whether it is anything like a constant rule for the after-stupor to be less persistent and less prolonged than in simple epilepsy.

7. Many of the persons in whom *apoplexy* is a probable danger are of a sanguine and plethoric constitution, corpulent, with large heads, short necks, and full chests; but there are many who have none of these characteristics. Nearly all are considerably past the meridian of life. Nearly all present various evidences of a depressed or debilitated brain—such as headache, weight in the head, want of memory, want of firmness, vertigo, ringings in the ears, specks before the eyes, apathy, or irritability of temper.

The different forms of apoplexy are arranged in three classes. In the first, the patient at once sinks into profound and deep coma; in the second he gradually passes into this state, after an attack of acute pain in the head, with faintness and sickness; in the third, he suddenly becomes paralysed on one side of the body, without losing his consciousness.

In the first class of cases the patient at once sinks into a sleep, from which no shouting, or pinching, or shaking will serve to wake him; and in this state he lies like a person dead-drunk, with his face flushed, his pulse slow, strong, and labouring, especially in the carotids, and his breathing deep, slow, and snoring. If a limb be pinched, it does not stir; if it be lifted up and let go, it falls like a log. The eye is absolutely indifferent to light, and the dilated pupil remains motionless under the full glare of the sun. In this state of deep sleep the patient lies for some time, and then he slowly wakes to find his judgment damaged, his fancy dulled, his feelings unmanageable, and half his body benumbed and motionless. Or this dangerous sleep may deepen into the sounder sleep of death, in which case the flush on the cheek gives way to a ghastly lividity, the pulse becomes weak, frequent, and irregular, the respiration shallower and interrupted with frequent sighs and pauses, the skin dusky and bathed in cold and clammy perspiration, and, before long, death is ushered in, either with or without convulsion. In a case like this, convulsion is not a common occurrence, and when it happens it is, as we have said, in the period of collapse preceding death, and not during the period of vascular activity which marks the beginning of the fit.

Or a person may fall down suddenly in this death-like sleep without this flushing of the face, and the insensible and unconscious body may lie, cold, pale, comparatively pulseless, without any loud and snoring breathings, and—whatever the issue of the attack, whether fortunate or unfortunate—with scarcely a single sign of vascular reaction from the beginning to the end. It is also another mark of distinction between this form of the attack and the one just described, that convulsion may mark the beginning of the fit or that certain muscles may be scized upon with spasm. In other respects it is the same, and if convulsion happens at another time, it is shortly before death.

In the second class of cases, the fit begins with sudden and violent pain in the head, confusion of thought, faintness, perhaps sickness. Instead of being flushed and hot, the face is pale and ghastly, the pulse weak, frequent, and irregular, the breathings shallow and interrupted with frequent sighs and pauses. Instead of being perfectly relaxed, the limbs are agitated, rigid, or convulsed, in which latter case the mental faculties are suspended for the time. Then, after a short time, the pulse rallies, the heat returns, the mind begins to reassert

13 §

its sway, and even the power of walking may be recovered; but the headache, instead of passing off, becomes more and more oppressive, until it is forgotten in the feelings of confusion, drowsiness, and coma, which succeed presently, (the interval between the first attack of pain and the occurrence of coma may vary from a few minutes to several hours.) Then the face again becomes pale and ghastly, the pulse fails, the respiration resumes its interrupted and sighing character, a cold and clammy perspiration breaks out all over the body, and the patient dies. In some of these cases death is ushered in by convulsion.

In the third class of cases, one side of the body is suddenly palsied and the power of speech destroyed, but without any corresponding loss of consciousness. The patient sees and hears and feels, thoughts also and memories arise in his mind; but he is stunned and bewildered. He only half apprehends the nature of the evil which has befallen him. In some cases, this state of things may continue for some time with little or no change, and then the patient may gradually sink from exhaustion or more speedily from coma. In other cases the mind may regain a great deal of what it had lost, and the palsy may gradually pass off—a change in which the leg is liberated before the arm, and the power of feeling before the power of motion.

In other cases, again, life is prolonged for a considerable time, and the only change is a state of contraction in the palsied muscles, of which more will have to be said presently. In cases like these there may be violent agitation at the beginning, but true epileptiform convulsion is not met with, except occasionally in the state of coma or collapse preceding death.

Now hæmorrhage may take place into the substance of the hemispheres, into the ventricles, or into the cavity of the arachnoid surrounding the brain, and different symptoms mark these different lesions, though as yet the nature of the difference cannot be determined with sufficient exactness. Premonitory symptoms, such as pain in the head, dulness, drowsiness—evidences of congestion—are said to be less common before hæmorrhage into the substance of the brain than before the other two forms of hæmorrhage. It is said that convulsion and muscular rigidity are much less common in hæmorrhage into the substance of the brain than in the other two forms of the disease. It is said, also, that coma is less profound and more slowly developed, and that paralysis is less general and complete in hæmorrhage into the cavity of the arachnoid external to the brain than in hæmorrhage into the ventricles. At any rate, there can be little doubt that ventricular apoplexy is the most formidable form of the malady.

But there is some uncertainty in these rules, and a review of many cases would rather seem to lead to the conclusion that the manner of the attack, the depth of the coma, and the extent of the paralysis, are determined by the quantity of blood effused and the suddenness of the effusion rather than by the site of the mischief—at least by the site simply. And certainly it is more than difficult to connect particular symptoms with injury to particular parts of the brain. Andral, for example, has disproved the idea that paralysis of the arm is specially connected with hæmorrhage into or upon the *corpus striatum,* and that paralysis of the leg has any necessary connexion with hæmorrhage into or upon the *thalamus opticus;* and Cruvelhier has shown very distinctly that loss of speech does not necessarily imply hæmorrhage into the anterior lobes.

— Now epileptiform convulsion cannot be said to be a frequent phenomenon in apoplexy; but if it does occur, it occurs at the times and under the circumstances which have been mentioned. The most frequent time for its occurrence is in the period of collapse preceding death. With respect to the convulsion itself, there is nothing at all peculiar.

8. *Inflammation of the brain* may affect the membranes or substance of this organ. The term

meningitis is restricted to inflammation of the pia-mater, which inflammation is indeed infinitely more important and far more common than inflammation of the two other membranes—the arachnoid and the dura-mater. The terms cerebritis or encephalitis, meningo-cerebritis, phrenitis, are used to express inflammation of the substance of the brain. Almost invariably the membranes, as well as the substance, are affected, and very often, if not generally, the membranes are affected primarily. Indeed, it is very questionable whether the membranes can be affected without implicating the subjacent portions of the brain; and it is not less questionable whether " our knowledge," (we quote from Abercrombie,) " is sufficiently matured to enable us to say *with confidence* what symptoms indicate inflammation of the substance of the brain as distinguished from that of the membranes."

(a.) *Meningitis* may be subdivided into three forms—the simple, the tubercular, and the rheumatic; and it will perhaps elucidate the history of the convulsion arising in this affection to observe this three-fold division.

Simple meningitis is the form which happens in healthy individuals. It begins with the precursory symptoms of fever—rigors, paleness of skin, cutis anserina, headache, depression, confusion, drowsiness, vomiting—often vomiting repeated many times.

Or, as Dr. Copland first pointed out, and especially in children, the initial rigors may be exaggerated into epileptiform convulsion. Then follow rapidly the symptoms of high febrile reaction, and the pulse becomes hard and frequent, the breathing irregular and oppressed, the skin hot, particularly over the head, the face flushed, the eye wild and ferretty. Along with these changes, the headache of the initiatory stage gives place to acute stabbing pain, and under these stabs the patient at times will shriek and scream from sheer agony. In some cases, a wild delirium takes the place of this acute pain, though this is doubted by Dr. Watson. All this time vomiting continues to be a distressing symptom. In this stage, which is called the first stage, the irritability is extreme, the pupil is contracted to the size of a pin's head, and the ear and eye are altogether impatient to sound or light. There may be strabismus; but in no case is there any marked prostration of strength. This stage continues for two or three days, and then the delirium calms down into quiet muttering, the headache ceases to be tormenting, or ceases altogether, the morbid sensitiveness passes off, the fever dies out. In losing its force the pulse becomes weak, small, irregular, or intermittent, and always very variable, at one moment slow, at the next frequent; and coincidently with this change in the pulse the respiration becomes irregular and interrupted with frequent sighs and pauses. As the flush leaves the cheek, the eye and ear cease to be impatient to light and sound, the pupil passes out of the contracted state, oscillates, and then becomes dilated and immovable, the countenance puts on a ghastly and cadaverous expression, the limbs give up their warmth, the whole body drips with cold and clammy perspiration, the restlessness of the first stage gives place to muscular tremblings or twitchings, or (especially in children) epileptiform convulsion makes its appearance. Itself ushered in by the symptoms which have been mentioned, the convulsion may usher in a state of fatal comatose prostration, in which, without cessation, convulsion may follow convulsion until the end. Or, without the convulsion, the muttering following the early delirium may quieten down into coma, and coma into death—an event which is occasionally hastened by the exhausting involuntary motions which have taken the place of the obstinate constipation of the early stage of the malady.

When the meningitis affects the base of the brain, there is, as a rule, less fever, less delirium, a greater disposition to convulsion, and a more speedy development of coma; but it is not possible to insist very positively upon the significance of these differences.

Tubercular meningitis, or that form which happens in scrofulous subjects, and generally in scrofulous children, is for the most part insidious in its course, and the symptoms are at times extremely vague. The acute stage of fever, with its wild delirium, distressing headache, and impatience to light or sound, are altogether wanting. There is enough pain to banish refreshing sleep, and now and then, particularly at night, there may be a pang so sharp as to provoke a scream. There may also be a little light-headedness in the evening or at night. The pulse is very variable, now quick, now slow, rising in frequency when the patient assumes a sitting or erect posture, and falling again when he lies down; and in the evening there may be some disposition to faint hectic excitement. The respiration is irregular, unequal, sighing. If unchecked, indeed, the patient rapidly and almost silently sinks into a state of collapse and coma, and not unfrequently he is seized with an epileptiform convulsion before we can bring ourselves to think that a serious disease is in progress. In cases like these, where the symptoms set in insidiously, convulsion would seem to happen less frequently at the commencement than in the period of collapse preceding death —at the time, that is to say, when the pulse is altogether without power, and when all cerebral action is being rapidly extinguished in coma—but it may happen at an earlier period. In any case, however, the convulsion is not associated with anything like feverish activity of the circulation. Indeed, the disease may be said to be without fever from beginning to end.

Rheumatic meningitis arises occasionally in the course of acute articular rheumatism, and the sufferers from it are generally weak and exhausted. The acute pain in the head, which is one of the symptoms, appears to have been translated from the limbs, for these limbs, whose least motion had been attended with great suffering, are now dashed about in all directions. Or, furious delirium may take the place of the pain. Indeed, the principal symptoms are acute pain in the head or furious delirium, followed rapidly, if their course be unfortunate, by drowsiness, coma and convulsions, paralysis and death. There is little febrile excitement from the beginning, and what little there is has died out before the occurrence of the convulsion; and there is less evidence of inflammatory action in the membranes after death,—indeed, such evidence is frequently wanting altogether.

(*b.*) *Cerebritis* is divided into two forms—general and partial.

General cerebritis (encephalitis, meningo-cerebritis, phrenitis), is commonly mixed up with a greater or less degree of meningitis, and any active delirium, or acute pain, or feverish excitement, would appear to be owing to this complication. Dulness, rapidly passing through drowsiness into coma, would seem to be the most characteristic phenomenon in uncomplicated cerebritis. Instead of the agonizing pain of simple meningitis, the headache is dull, oppressive, deep-seated; instead of a morbid impatience, even in darkness and silence, the eye and ear are almost indifferent to light and sound; vomiting is a frequent and distressing symptom; and obstinate constipation is always present. The pulse, at first, is slow, but presently becomes variable, and readily influenced by changes of posture; the respiration, also, is variable and suspirious, or presently becomes so. Each hour, indeed, the pulse loses in power, more sighs and pauses are mixed up in the respirations, and after the last semblance of excitement has passed off, and when the deepness of the drowsiness shows that coma is at hand, with its companion—death, then, in all probability, the frame is shaken with one or two paroxysms of convulsion.

Partial cerebritis ("red softening," acute ramollissement), has even less febrile disturbance than general cerebritis, and its course is much slower. The mental faculties fail, the eyes become dim, the ears dull, the features torpid, the tongue trips, the power of moving and feeling depart from one side of the body, and at no distant date convulsion and coma supervene. The paralysis is often preceded by a rigid state of the muscles. There is, moreover, dull, fixed pain in the head, and achings in the limbs, particularly in those that are palsied; the head is somewhat hotter than it ought to be; and vertigo and vomiting are no unfrequent symptoms. The state of coma may pass off and recur again several times, apparently in consequence of the phenomena of congestion being mixed up with those of partial cerebritis; but at last there is an attack which does not pass off, and the patient sinks. In the course of the disease, and always in close connexion with the coma, there may be many epileptiform seizures.

9. The convulsion connected with *fever* arises at two distinct periods—at the onset and at the end of the disorder. That which happens at the onset is a common event in the fevers of children, particularly in smallpox; and it is an occasional event in the fevers of adults. Its antecedents, in all probability, have been failure of appetite, unrefreshing sleep, feebleness, want of spirit. Its immediate accompaniments are a sense of great feebleness or oppression, sickness or vomiting, paleness of the face, coldness of the hands and feet, cutis anserina, shivering or shuddering, headache, pain and sense of coldness in the back or limbs, a

feeble, soft, and fluctuating pulse, a respiration short, accelerated, and interrupted with frequent sighs. These symptoms continue for a time varying from one to twelve hours, and then coldness gives place to unnatural heat, and the pulse becomes full and bounding, or wiry and incompressible,—in a word, that change takes place which is known as the establishment of fever. Under ordinary circumstances rigor or shuddering is the extent of the muscular disturbance attendant upon the onset of fever; but in some instances the rigor is, as it were, exaggerated into convulsion, in which case the depression and oppression of the primary period of collapse have been more marked, the depression under these circumstances amounting to prostration, and the oppression to stupor. In a word, the convulsion which is occasionally attendant upon the onset of fever is as distinctly related to the period of collapse preceding the outbreak of fever, and as distinctly separated from the period of febrile reaction, as is the rigor of which it is the representative.

And so also with the convulsion which may come on towards the close of fever. The true febrile reaction is over. The pulse is weak and thready, the hand frigid, the body is already clammy with the sweats of death, the face is putting on the ghastliness of the grave, the muttering remains of a previous delirium are upon the point of dying out, and then—when the hand of death is already upon the heart, and the fire of life flickers faintly among embers that are well-nigh cold—the twitchings of the muscles may be exaggerated into convulsion. These are the circumstances attending upon the convulsion which may happen towards the end of fever.

10. Epileptiform convulsion is often brought about by the retention of some of the constituents of urine in the blood, and occasionally by the retention of some of the elements of the biliary excretion, and the history of the convulsion arising under these circumstances is not at all obscure.

— The constituents of *urine may be retained* in the blood in Bright's disease of the kidney, in cholera and typhoid fever, after scarlet fever, and occasionally during pregnancy, as when the emulgent veins are pressed upon by the growing uterus. The causes of retention may, indeed, vary considerably; but, however different the cause, the system is brought substantially into the same state before the convulsion happens.

In a case of Bright's disease, where the history of the convulsion is perhaps defined most clearly, the attention is first arrested by unmistakeable evidences of debility and emaciation, the skin is pale, and in certain parts, as about the eyelids and ankles, it is puffy and pits on pressure. Appetite is wanting, ammonia is present in the breath, as may readily be seen by breathing on a glass rod which has been dipped in hydrochloric acid, a pale yellow fluid containing ammonia is occasionally ejected from the stomach, diarrhœa is, it may be, an urgent symptom, and the urine is scanty, loaded with albumen or casts, and wanting in a proper quantity of urea. The patient, moreover, is drowsy, stupid, listless, despondent, seeing and hearing with some difficulty, drawling in his speech, tripping in his gait, palsied in one or other of his limbs to a greater or less extent, and frequently suffering from annoying cramps. Each day these symptoms are aggravated, the drowsiness becoming more oppressive, the bodily strength more exhausted, and when this aggravation has reached a certain point, convulsion and coma make their appearance. This state of coma is peculiar in not being complete. The patient breathes stertorously, and, if let alone, appears to be dead to all within and around him, but he starts at a loud noise, or withdraws his hand if it be pinched or pricked, and for a moment the stertor ceases. Occasionally, also, he may partially wake out of this comatose condition, and delirious mutterings may show that the brain has resumed some degree of action. The stertor, moreover, is peculiar in being set at a higher pitch than that which is heard in ordinary apoplexy. The epileptiform convulsions occurring under these circumstances are frequently, as a rule, not very severe, and they often alternate with rigidity of the limbs, which rigidity varies in amount and position, and is often increased by any attempt to move the parts. These convulsions may recur several times: they are close companions of the coma; and like the coma, they are connected with a state which differs very little from collapse—a state of which a pale and cadaverous face and cold extremities are among the signs.

— Epileptiform convulsion is not a common consequence of *retention of bile,* and where it does occur it is in a comatose or semi-comatose state, which is very similar to that which is brought on by retention of urine. At an earlier stage of the malady there may have been high fever and active delirium, but all signs of true excitement have passed off, and the condition is closely akin to collapse and coma when the convulsion happens. In a case of this kind the jaundiced skin will serve to point out the seat of the mischief.

11. The children which have any difficulty in cutting their teeth are undoubtedly delicate rather than strong. Their gums are swollen, tender, and painful, they are fretful and disposed to cry, their

sleep is short and disturbed with starts, and they suffer in all probability from vomiting and diarrhœa as well as from want of appetite. A little later, when they have become exhausted by pain and want of sleep, and wasted by want of food and diarrhœa or vomiting, fretfulness and wakefulness change into drowsiness, the pulse becomes excessively weak, and under these circumstances convulsion may happen. Or, instead of drowsiness thus coming on with little or no fever, it may have been preceded by symptoms of cerebral inflammation or determination with high fever; in which case the convulsion may occur, as in ordinary fever, either in the initial stage of rigor, or in the period of collapse and coma which comes on after the state of feverish or inflammatory excitement has altogether passed off.

Where convulsion is referred to "irritation" in the alimentary canal, the blame is often thrown upon worms, and worms are often present. But if worms are not present there are always some other evidences of constitutional debility, bodily or mental. Very often the appetite fails, the breath becomes offensive, the pulse quick, the bowels confined and teased with aches and gripes; and these fits of febrile disturbance, brought on for the most part by the presence of undigested food, leave the patient jaded, irritable, perhaps drowsy, emaciated, and liable to convulsion. Or, instead of simple irritability and drowsiness, there may have been more active fever and delirium ending in a comatose condition and a liability to convulsion. In either case the convulsion happens under similar circumstances—a brain that is either drówsy or semi-comatose and a body that is exhausted and probably emaciated.

Nor is there anything peculiar in the history of the convulsion which is not unfrequently connected with menstruation, or pregnancy, or parturition, and of which irritation in the uterus is often regarded as a cause.

In epileptiform convulsion connected with the menstrual periods it often happens that the fit occurs at the end of these periods, when mind and body are alike exhausted by pain or loss of blood. It often happens, also, that the persons who suffer in this manner possess all the mental and bodily characteristics which belong to epileptic or hysterical patients, and that the attacks themselves have nothing to distinguish them from epileptic or hysterical attacks.

A similar remark may also be made with respect to the convulsion which occasionally happens during the course of pregnancy. For this convulsion may be either epileptic or hysterical; or it may be brought about by pressure upon the emulgent veins, in which case the general condition is analogous to that which has been pointed out when speaking of the convulsion connected with urinæmia.

And so also with the convulsion which occasionally happens during labour. It may be an attack of ordinary epilepsy or hysteria, or it may be brought about by loss of blood or by sheer nervous exhaustion. In the case of flooding, the face and tongue are blanched, the hand is frigid, the body bathed in cold sweat, the pupil dilated, the sight swimming and dim, the ear stunned with ringing and booming noises, the head racked with throbbing pain, the limbs incessantly tossed about, the trunk agitated with frequent shudderings and shocks, the stomach straining with constant efforts at retching and vomiting, the thoughts indistinct and in a constant whirl, the pulse fluttering or imperceptible, the breathing a continued sigh or gasp. With such accompaniments and after the last trace of mental action has died out, convulsion happens. In the other case, where convulsion comes on in the course of labour without flooding, the patient has been exhausted by the pain and effort; straining continually, apoplexy may be the result of the impeded circulation in the brain; or pain, delirium, drowsiness, coma, may sufficiently show the kind of mischief that is going on within the skull. Now it is in this state of drowsiness or coma, when all cerebral action is annihilated or upon the verge of annihilation, and when the bodily powers are upon the point of yielding in the struggle, that the convulsion happens, of which mention is now made. The convulsion itself is often as violent as the worst form of epilepsy, and the attendant suffocation is often very marked, and in this respect it differs from the convulsion of flooding, where the convulsion is most generally less marked and less prolonged.

Nor is there anything peculiar in the history of the convulsion which occasionally arises in the fortnight following delivery; for, if this convulsion is not simply epileptic or hysterical, it is connected with the last stage of puerperal fever, and the attendant symptoms are the same as those which accompany the convulsion happening towards the close of any fever.

And in those cases of convulsion which are referred to "irritation" of a sexual character, the same history is sufficiently obvious—mental exhaustion, accompanied by more or less bodily exhaustion, of which so much has been said already, the fits happening in or near the times of greatest exhaustion.

12. Convulsion is a frequent symptom where the *moribund state* is brought about by the loss of blood, and in this case the collateral circumstances

are those which have just been described as occurring in flooding. Convulsion may also be present when death is caused, not by loss of blood, but by loss of the power which carries on the circulation, as in cases of "shock," or in poisoning by hydrocyanic acid and certain other poisons; and in these cases, the surface is cold, the circulation and respiration are almost at a stand-still, and all mental action is altogether annihilated when the convulsion happens.

Convulsion, also, is the natural accompaniment of death by suffocation, whether sudden or gradual When the lungs are suddenly deprived of fresh air, the face and neck immediately become "black and full of blood," the veins stand out like thick cords, the eyes appear to be starting from their sockets. In the first few instants there is an agonizing struggle for breath; in the instants following the symptoms are delirium of a pleasant character (so it is said), vertigo, loss of consciousness, convulsion, relaxation, death. The pulse, at first feeble, becomes stronger and fuller as the turmoil proceeds; and, at the time when the suffocation is well nigh complete, the main arteries may throb with considerable force. After this it fails rapidly; but it may be felt at the wrist for a short time after the patient is apparently dead.

In cases, where the suffocation is brought about

slowly, as in pulmonary congestion or inflammation and in effusion into the pleura, the distressing efforts to breathe, the dusky or livid countenance, the giddy feelings, the delirious thoughts, are some of the symptoms which show the terrible prostration of the vital powers, and, when convulsion comes, it is hand-in-hand with fatal prostration and coma. In cases where slow suffocation is the effect of the suspension of the action of the great nervous centres, as in apoplexy, the distressing efforts to breathe, the giddy feelings and the delirious thoughts are not present, but the dusky and lurid countenance, the slow, irregular, and stertorous breathings, and the fluttering pulse, are sufficient to show that there is a prostration deeper than that of mere coma when the convulsion happens.

The pathology of epileptiform convulsion.

(*a.*) *The pathology of epileptiform convulsion as deduced from a consideration of the vascular system.*

In a case of general epileptiform convulsion the state of the circulation is as far removed from anything like excitement as it is in epilepsy. There is, indeed, the same failure of the pulse at the commencement of the fit, and the same state of positive suffocation during the fit. In a case of partial epileptiform convulsion the state of the circulation is one in which the phenomena of extreme prostration are mixed up with those of suffocation. In any case, the pulse is scarcely to be felt at the beginning of the paroxysm, and everything shows that the circulation is at the very lowest ebb; and if the pulse acquires any semblance of power as the paroxysm proceeds, the dusky and livid colour of the face, the interrupted breathings, and other unequivocal signs of suffocation, afford sufficient proof that this phenomenon is due, not to the increased injection of red blood into the arteries, but to the resistance which the unaërated blood encounters in passing through the systemic capillaries.

Nor is there any evidence of a contrary character in the vascular antecedents of epileptiform convulsion, for in those cases in which the malady is of an inflammatory or febrile character, it will be seen that the fit occurs, either in the period of collapse which precedes the development of the inflammation or fever, or else in the period of collapse which comes after the dying out of this fever or inflammation.

1. In *chronic softening of the brain* the habitual coldness of the hands and feet, the weakened and perhaps degenerated heart, the cord-like arteries, are among the signs which show the innate weakness of the circulation—a weakness to which fever or inflammation are alike uncongenial.

2. In *chronic meningitis,* as might be expected from the state of weakness and exhaustion which is so generally present, the pulse for the most part is quick, weak, and much affected by changes of posture. There may be some faint evidences of hectic excitement in the evening, when the cheeks flush, the eyes shine, and the aching head becomes a little hotter than it was before; but this faint excitement is not sufficient to raise the pulse to a normal pitch of activity. In no case, indeed, is this faint excitement of the circulation a marked and conspicuous phenomenon, and in the majority of instances it is scarcely sufficient to impart even a semblance of power to the weak and feverless pulse. And if there is little vascular excitement in chronic meningitis, there is if possible less in the form of disease which is known under the name of *chronic hydrocephalus.*

3. In *tumour of the brain* the pulse is quick, weak, irritable, fluctuating, or, if it is not, it will be so as soon as pain, want of sleep, and despondency —common symptoms of tumour—have had time to bear their natural fruit of weakness and exhaustion.

4. In *induration of the brain,* such as is met with in lead poisoning, the phenomena presented by the circulation differ very little, if at all, from those which occur in advanced stages of simple epilepsy,

and any difference there may be is one which indicates a state still more fully removed from fever.

5. In *atrophy of the brain,* as in simple epilepsy, there is no evidence of anything like excitement in the circulation.

6. In *congestion of the brain* the head and face are congested and dusky, the lips purple, the jugulars full, the pulse and respiration slow and laboured, the hands and feet habitually colder than the head. There are, indeed, many evident signs which show that the circulation is not carried on with proper vigour, and which appear to point to imperfect arterialization of the blood as one cause of this defect.

7. In *apoplexy* the convulsion is most apt to happen at the end rather than at the beginning of the period of coma, when the purpled lips and the inadequate breathings show that the respiratory changes are rapidly failing. Or, if it happens at the beginning, it is in those forms in which the condition of the circulation at the time is more akin to collapse than anything else, and not in those forms in which there is an excited pulse and strong determination of blood to the head.

8. In *inflammation of the brain* the condition of the circulation is not uniformly the same at all times, but this condition, as will be seen by reflect-

ing on what has been already said, varies little with respect to the convulsion.

(*a.*) *Simple meningitis* begins with paleness of the skin, a feeble depressed pulse, cutis anserina, vomiting, rigors, perhaps convulsion. Then follow rapidly the symptoms of high febrile reaction and cerebral inflammation—the pulse becoming hard and frequent, the breathings irregular and oppressed, the skin, particularly the skin of the head, hot and burning. These symptoms of high febrile reaction and inflammation continue for two or three days, and then give place to an opposite state of things, in which the pulse loses its force and becomes weak, small, irregular, and the breathings are interrupted with frequent sighs and pauses. Or if at this time the pulse retains any degree of resistance, it is evident from the dusky colour of the skin and the suspirious and laboured respiration, that the whole of this resistance is not due to the injection of arterial blood into the artery. Now it is in this stage of collapse which follows the period of inflammatory and febrile excitement, or else in the stage of collapse which precedes the febrile and inflammatory excitement, and never during the actual period of excitement, that the convulsion happens. And this rule is constant. Indeed, the history of simple meningitis shows most conclusively that

14 §

vascular excitement is as incompatible with convulsion, as it is with rigor or subsultus.

In *tubercular meningitis* the pulse is weak and variable from the very first, now quick, now comparatively slow, rising in frequency when the head is raised from the pillow, and falling upon lying down again; and from the very first, the respiration is irregular, unequal, and interrupted with frequent sighs and pauses. For some time there may be some little disturbance of a hectic character, particularly in the evening; but this soon comes to an end, and the prostrate pulse forgets to put on even this faint semblance of fever. In some cases, there may indeed be a short stage of fever, and something like cerebral inflammation, especially in young children; but as a rule, the symptoms are altogether of a passive, non-febrile, non-inflammatory character. In any case, however, the convulsion is connected with an extremely depressed state of the circulation, and never with a state of febrile and inflammatory excitement, if there be such a state.

In *rheumatic meningitis*, also, there is little or no febrile excitement from the beginning, and the pulse has become feverless and utterly weak before the convulsion happens.

(*b.*) In *general cerebritis* the pulse, at first slow,

soon becomes variable and readily affected by changes of posture: the respiration, also, is very variable and suspirious. From the first, indeed, there is scarcely any fever, and little heat of head, except the phenomena of cerebritis are mixed up with those of simple meningitis; but if such symptoms are present, they soon pass off, and give place to symptoms of slow sinking—a state in which hour by hour the breathing is more interrupted with sighs and pauses, and the pulse more powerless, unless it may derive some fictitious power from the difficult circulation of imperfectly arterialized blood, in which case the dusky countenance and the purple lips will show very clearly that the vessel is not altogether filled with arterial blood.

In *partial cerebritis* there is even less febrile disturbance than there is in general cerebritis, and at no stage of the malady is there anything like increased vascular action.

9. The immediate antecedents of the epileptiform convulsion which may attend upon the onset of *fever*, are paleness of the face, coldness of the hands and feet, a feeble, soft, and fluctuating pulse, a respiration that is short, accelerated, and interrupted with frequent sighs. The immediate antecedents of the convulsion which may attend upon the end of fever, are a weak and thready pulse, a frigid hand, and lungs too much gorged with blood to allow of

any proper respiration—a state in which the febrile reaction has long since died out, and the hand of death is already upon the heart. The convulsion, indeed, takes the place either of rigor or subsultus, and like these forms of muscular disturbance, it is associated, not with the state of febrile excitement, but with a state of depression which is as much below the natural standard as the state of febrile excitement is above that standard.

10. The convulsion which may follow *retention of urine,* is preceded by cold hands and feet, by a retarded and sighing respiration, by a weak pulse, or if at all otherwise, the evidences of defective respiration are sufficient to show that the pulse derives a fictitious strength from the difficult circulation of imperfectly arterialized blood. And so, also, with the convulsion connected with the *retention of bile,* for before the convulsion makes its appearance, all evidences of high fever and active determination of blood to the head have died out, and the symptoms of positive sinking have taken their place.

11. In the convulsion connected with *dentition,* there may have been little or no previous fever, and by quick degrees the pulse may have become excessively weak. Or there may have been symptoms of cerebral inflammation with high fever, and after them a state bordering very closely upon collapse.

In any case, the immediate antecedents of the fit are indicative of great vascular depression—great vascular depression brought on slowly without any very obvious fever or determination of blood to the head, or else that which precedes or succeeds active fever and determination. And so likewise with that convulsion which is connected with *worms,* or other sources of irritation in the alimentary canal, for if there have been any fits of febrile disturbance, these fits have died out, and left the patient, not only feverless, but pale and chilly. Nor is it otherwise with those forms of convulsion which are referred to irritation in the *uterus.* In the convulsion connected with menstruation, the circulation is such as has been described in hysteria or epilepsy when the attack is hysteric or epileptic in its character; and a similar remark applies to several of the convulsions which may happen in the course of pregnancy. In the convulsion of flooding, the face and even the tongue is blanched, the hand frigid, the body bathed in cold sweat, the pulse fluttering and scarcely to be detected, the breathing a continuous sigh or gasp. In the convulsion occurring in labour, in which there has been no flooding, the head is often greatly congested, and the aëration of the blood is seriously interfered with, partly as a consequence of the way in which the lungs sympathise with the semi-comatose brain, and partly because the regular expansions of the chest are interfered with by the constant efforts at straining. In such a case the pulse may be full, but if so, the venous colour of the lips will show that this fulness is due to the impediment which an imperfectly arterialized blood opposes to its circulation through the systemic capillaries. In the convulsion which may happen during puerperal fever, the vascular antecedents are the same as those which may happen towards the end of any fever. And lastly, the condition of the circulation before the convulsion which is referred to "irritation" of a sexual character, if it differs at all from that which is met with in ordinary epilepsy, only differs in being one of still deeper depression.

12. Nor is there any trace of vascular excitement before the convulsion which may happen in the *moribund state*. In the convulsion attending death by hæmorrhage or asthenia, the blanched face and tongue, the frigid hand, the sighing or gasping respiration, the faltering pulse, are signs which require no comment; and in the convulsion attending death by speedy or gradual suffocation, the state of things is equally opposed to the idea of vascular excitement, for how can vascular excitement and a state of suffocation be compatible conditions?

— In a word, there is no instance in which epileptiform convulsion can be supposed to have any connexion with an excited state of the vascular system, and there are many instances in which the circulation is removed almost as far as possible from such a state: and the only conclusion which can be drawn from these facts is one which harmonizes with the physiological premises and with the previous conclusions respecting the kindred questions in pathology.

(*b.*) *The pathology of epileptiform convulsion as deduced from a consideration of the phenomena connected with the nervous system.*

In a case of general epileptiform convulsion the mental faculties are suspended as completely as they are in epilepsy. The dilated pupil remains immoveable under the brightest light, the ear is deaf to the loudest noise, and when the patient recovers, if he does recover, his memory is an absolute blank as to everything that happened during the fit. In partial epileptiform convulsion, such as occurs not unfrequently in chronic softening and tumour of the brain, as in partial epileptic convulsion, the mental faculties may not be altogether suspended, and the memory is occasionally able to recall some of the circumstances attending the fit. In the case of general epileptiform convulsion, therefore, the condition of the mind is evidently one of *inaction,* and not of action. This is evidently so. Nor can there be any doubt that the state of the mind is one of comparative inaction in partial epileptiform convulsion, for the utter bewilderment, the inability to collect and control the thoughts, the trepidation, and the want of control over the muscles, are all signs that cannot be misinterpreted.

It would seem, also, that the inaction of the brain must extend to other faculties besides the mental faculties, and that the brain is not less inactive than every other centre of nervous action, for (to repeat the argument already used on more than one occasion) it is not easy to believe that any but the lowest degree of action is compatible with a circulation in which the aëration of the blood is altogether or in great measure suspended, or which is balancing upon the very verge of syncope. And, certainly, the aëration of the blood is as completely suspended by suffocation, or the circulation as nearly brought to a stand-still, in epileptiform convulsion as in epilepsy.

Nor is there anything contradictory to this conclusion in the facts which remain to be mentioned.

1. In *chronic softening of the brain* the fits are preceded by unquestionable and often very marked impairment of the mental faculties, and in some cases the mind may be a total wreck. Dulness

steadily changing into drowsiness, and drowsiness deepening into coma; these are the most conspicuous features of this sad condition. The brain, also, is blighted, not inflamed. It is pallid, whiter than it ought to be, deficient in red spots, and in parts softer than natural; and the softened substance when examined microscopically is found to consist of broken-down brain-tissue, with a greater or less number of cells containing oil, and sometimes reddened with blood-corpuscles (for hæmorrhage is a common consequence of softening), but without any of the products of inflammation, such as exudations or pus-corpuscles.

2. Impairment of the mental faculties, progressively increasing, is also a prominent symptom in *chronic meningitis*, and this impairment would seem to be more marked by peevishness, impatience, fidgetiness, and a disposition to delirium, than by dulness. The mind wanders a little in the evening or at night, and not unfrequently this wandering may settle down into insanity. Or there may be no positive symptoms of any kind. After death the principal sign of disorder is an effusion of serum beneath the arachnoid or into the ventricles, and this is often the only sign. In some instances there may be some congestion of the pia mater, or some evidences of tubercular degeneration in this membrane and in the contiguous parts of the brain,

but, as a rule, the appearances are altogether negative. Indeed, in some instances, where the quantity of effused fluid is large, as in chronic hydrocephalus, the brain has a blanched, bloodless appearance, and the effused fluid is much less rich in solid constituents than the serum of the blood—a fact which is somewhat calculated to show that inflammation has had no share in its production.

3. In the majority of cases of *tumour* the intelligence does not appear to suffer in any very marked manner, and when it is otherwise it is owing in some degree at least to the presence of chronic meningitis. The pain, however, the want of sleep, the depression of spirits, all combine to exhaust the brain, and this exhaustion is shown by vagueness in the ideas, inability to fix the thoughts, and in various other ways. Nor is the pain which is usually so very distressing a symptom an objection to the idea that the brain is acting inefficiently in these cases. In many cases, indeed, pain in the head is a sign that the brain is insufficiently supplied with arterial blood, for it ceases and gives place to delirium when the arterial injection increases. And in some instances, at least, there is reason to believe that the nervous energy is *lessened* during pain. At any rate, Dr. Du Bois-Raymond has shown by means of the galvanometer that the "nerve-current" fails whenever the nerve

is treated in a way that will cause pain. These experiments, it is true, have only been tried upon the nerves of frogs, and the influence tested by the galvanometer is simply electrical; but still there is no reason for supposing that the nerves of frogs are essentially different from other nerves, and there is much reason for believing that electricity and nervous influence are connected in such a way that the condition of the one may be looked upon as an index of the state of the other; and if so, then the experiment in question may be supposed to furnish *some* reason for believing that pain may be as much a sign of want of action in the sentient nerve as spasm is a sign of want of action in the muscular fibre. Be this as it may in other instances, however, it must be difficult to appeal to the pain as a sign of over-action of the brain in tumour, for the symptoms during life and the appearances after death are alike opposed to such a conclusion.

4. In *induration of the brain,* such as results from lead-poisoning, there is as little evidence of any excitement in the mental faculties as in epilepsy, probably less; and the condition of the brain after death affords no countenance to the idea of inflammation, for the brain is harder, darker in colour, drier, more bloodless than it ought to be.

5. In cases of *atrophy of the brain,* where the condition is congenital, the probabilities are that

the patient is idiotic as well as epileptic. In cases of hypertrophy of the brain, which cases are occasionally met with in children, while the bones are sufficiently yielding to allow the necessary expansion of the organ, the patients have not had any other inconvenience beyond the deformity—a faint argument, possibly, that want of brain, and therefore want of cerebral action, had really to do with the convulsion which would seem to be a constant phenomenon in atrophy of the brain.

6. A person suffering from *congestion of the brain* is less "bright" than he was, his conceptions are wanting in clearness, he is deficient in the power of attention and application, his sight is dim, his hearing dull and perplexed with rumbling sounds, he is drowsy, and feelings of weight in the head and pain are familiar troubles. Everything, indeed, indicates an oppressed and inactive brain.

7. In *apoplexy* the mental antecedents are those of congestion or softening, and not of inflammation as such. There would indeed appear to be a strange absence of inflammatory tendency in the brain in apoplexy, and if there are any evidences of inflammatory action around the clot it will generally be found that this action was anterior to the hæmorrhage in point of time—that, in fact, the blood has escaped in consequence of a previously softened state of brain. It is possible, also, that an argu-

ment in favour of a tendency directly opposed to the idea of inflammation may be found in the fact, pointed out by MM. Andral and Gavarral, that the blood is deficient in fibrine in apoplexy, for if the effect of inflammation be to increase the amount of fibrine contained in the blood, it may be supposed that a deficiency of fibrine is indicative of a tendency which is the reverse of inflammation.

8. Nor is there the least reason to believe that any over-action of the brain is concerned in bringing about the convulsion which is connected with *inflammation of the brain.*

(*a.*) In *simple meningitis,* convulsion may attend upon the very onset of the disorder, and in this case it is in the period of collapse which ushers in the true inflammatory stage—a period of which the mental signs are depression, confusion, perhaps drowsiness. Or convulsion may attend upon the period of final prostration which follows the true inflammatory stage—a period in which the mind is rapidly sinking towards a state of coma. Convulsion may occur at one or other of these times, but it never occurs in the true inflammatory stage. It never occurs, that is to say, when the pupil is contracted to the size of a pin's-head, when the impatience of the eye and ear is scarcely to be quietened by absolute darkness or silence, and while there is agonizing pain in the head or fierce delirium.

In *tubercular meningitis* the acute pain, the wild delirium, the intolerance of light or sound, which mark the outburst of simple meningitis are wanting, and the course of the disease is insidious. In cases such as these, where the symptoms set in stealthily, the usual period for the convulsion is after the brain and the system generally have given many unequivocal signs of exhaustion. In other cases, where the course of the disease is less insidious—where, that is to say, there is more febrile and inflammatory disturbance—there may be convulsion at the onset of the disorder, as well as at the time when all febrile and inflammatory disturbance has calmed down and left the system in a jaded and exhausted state. In these cases, indeed, as in cases of simple meningitis, there may be convulsion in the period of initial collapse or rigor preceding the establishment of the febrile or inflammatory disturbance. At best, however, the evidences of such disturbance are feebly marked, both during life and after death. Indeed, the name inflammation is as little applicable to this affection as it is to pulmonary phthisis, for when the diseased products are examined microscopically, they are found to consist, not of the products of inflammation, but of the well-known elements of ordinary tubercle.

In *rheumatic meningitis* the convulsion observes the same rule, occurring either in the initial period of rigor or collapse preceding the accession of the violent pain and delirium, or else after the period of excitement has died out and left the patient drowsy and comatose.

(*b.*) In *general cerebritis* anything like wild delirium, or acute pain in the head, is absent, unless it is complicated with meningitis, and the characteristic state is dulness and drowsiness, rapidly passing into typhoid prostration. In *partial cerebritis* the course of the disease is less rapid, and the downward progress may be interrupted by pauses of longer or shorter duration, but in other respects its characters are the same. From beginning to end, in either case, there are no evidences of an excited state of the brain to be gathered from the mental phenomena, or certainly there are no such evidences at the time the convulsions make their appearance.

9. In *fever* convulsion may precede the establishment of the febrile excitement, in which case the mental state is one of great depression, oppression, prostration, stupefaction. In other words, it may occur in the initial period of collapse or rigor. Or it may occur in the final period of prostration, when a few incoherent mutterings are the only traces of the previous delirium, when the last traces of mental action are rapidly succumbing to the drowsiness of approaching death. It may, occur at one or other of these times, but not during the active period of the fever.

10. In epileptiform convulsion depending upon *retention of urine* the patient before the attack is drowsy, stupid, listless, despondent, his eyesight dim, his hearing dull, his speech drawling; and in convulsion depending upon *retention of bile* delirium is at an end, and the drowsiness is well-nigh comatose before the time for the attack has arrived.

11. In difficult *dentition* the brain is exhausted by pain and want of sleep, and drowsiness has taken the place of fretfulness and wakefulness before the time for the fit has arrived; or if there has been any cerebral inflammation or determination, the fit follows the rule which has been already laid down. In *worms*, and in other forms of " irritation " in the alimentary canal, the mind as well as the body are far from being braced up to the proper pitch of health, and the patient is jaded, irritable, and drowsy. In the convulsion occurring at the times of menstruation or during pregnancy, the mental state will be found to correspond with the state which is characteristic of epilepsy or hysteria. In the convulsion of flooding the pupil is dilated, the thoughts are faint and incoherent, and before the tossings change into convulsion, the last trace of mental action has died out. In convulsion occurring during a labour in which there has been no flooding, the brain is exhausted by pain and straining, and upon the point of lapsing into a state of coma at the time

the convulsion happens. In the convulsion of puerperal fever the mental history is the same as the convulsion of ordinary fever; and in the convulsion which is referred especially to "irritation" of a sexual character, this history agrees in every respect with the history of hysteria or epilepsy.

Nor is it to be supposed that "morbid irritability" has any special part to play in these forms of convulsion, for after what has been already said, it is evident that such a property has less to do with the phenomenon of convulsion than inflammation.

12. And, lastly, there can be no doubt as to the condition of the brain connected with the *moribund state*. In death by hæmorrhage or asthenia, mental action fails *pari passu* with the flowing of the blood out of the vessels, or its stagnation in them, and the sufferer has become altogether insensible to pain and trouble before he is convulsed. And when death is brought about by suffocation, whether slowly or rapidly, it is no less certain that all mental action fails as the respiratory changes fail, and that no single trace of it remains when the time for the convulsion has arrived.

— Wherever epileptiform convulsion makes its appearance, therefore, the attack is preceded by some evident failure in mental energy, and in several instances this failure is almost or altogether complete. Nor is it possible to suppose that this state of inaction is confined to that part of the nervous system which is the scene of mental action, for it has been seen previously, that the attack is preceded by a depressed or oppressed state of circulation which involves a corresponding state of depression or oppression in the action of every part of the nervous system.

— In a word, there is nothing in the pathology of epileptiform convulsion, as deduced from a consideration of the phenomena connected with the nervous system, which is not in keeping with all the previous conclusions, physiological as well as pathological.

The treatment of epileptiform convulsion.

In cases where epileptiform convulsion is symptomatic of cerebral disease of a *chronic character*—chronic softening, chronic meningitis, tumour, induration, atrophy—the treatment called for would seem to agree in all its main features with that which is required in simple epilepsy.

In none of these cases does there appear to be any good reason why the patient should be put upon short commons. In chronic softening, indeed, it may be supposed that the disease, which is essentially atrophic, will gain ground if the diet be scanty and insufficient. It is of course necessary to avoid the risk of vascular fulness and possible hæmorrhage, by taking care that the diet does not err on the side of liberality; but of the two errors it would really seem that the patient is damaged less by a diet which is too liberal than by a diet which is insufficient. In chronic meningitis, a little abstinence may now and then be necessary, in consequence of slight fits of feverishness; but it must never be forgotten, that the part which inflammation has to play in this malady, is infinitely less important than that which is played by degeneration, and that an evident scrofulous taint is scarcely ever absent. It must never be forgotten, indeed, that the general history of the disorder is such as to demand a generous diet, if any inference is to be drawn from the history of other diseases in which the same taint is manifested. The same remarks are applicable, also, not only to tubercle of the brain, but also to cancer, for it is certain that both these maladies are likely to progress most rapidly where the system is low and ill-nourished. In both these cases of tumour, indeed, as well as in other cases of the kind, even in tumour of an aneurismal character, the exhaustion arising from pain and want of sleep and mental depression would seem to constitute a special call, not only for nourishment, but also for a fair allowance of stimulants. Nor is it more easy to suppose that induration of the brain or atrophy are reasons for enjoining a low diet.

In other respects, also, it would seem that the remarks respecting the arrangement of the diet and the adjustment of the habits, which were made when speaking of simple epilepsy, are still applicable to those cases of epileptiform convulsion depending upon chronic disease of the brain.

Nor is there any sufficient reason for supposing that any essential change is required in the general plan of treatment by medicines. In chronic meningitis, or in tumour of the brain, cod-liver oil may be the most suitable tonic; in tumour, moreover, the pain and want of sleep and depression of spirits may require the addition of morphia or of some other remedy of the kind; in induration of the brain from lead poisoning it may be necessary to follow out the plan suggested by M. Melsens, and give iodide of potassium before anything else can be done; in every case, indeed, there will be some special point which requires to be attended to; but there is no reason for supposing that the essential line of treatment will be different from that which has been laid down when speaking of simple epilepsy. And this remark applies to the treatment of the fit as well as to the treatment of the intervals between the fits.

— In cases where the epileptiform convulsion is symptomatic of disorder of an *acute character*, the practical question which must be decided before any other is whether the fit occurs at the beginning or at the close of the disorder. If at the beginning—as at the onset of fever or of certain forms of inflammation of the brain—little, in all probability, will have to be done, for the speedy establishment of the fever or inflammation will put an end to the convulsion, and prevent its recurrence for a time. If the fit occurs at the close of the disorder, the treatment of the convulsion resolves itself into the treatment of the disorder. Now, according to the premises, convulsion in itself is not a reason for the adoption of antiphlogistic measures. On the contrary, it is a phenomenon which would be likely to be brought about by anything which would exhaust the brain and nervous system; and therefore a question arises, whether the occurrence of convulsion at the end of certain disorders might not be prevented in some degree, by more carefully husbanding the strength of the patient during the active period of the disorder.

— In the routine treatment of *congestion of the brain and apoplexy,* bloodletting, purgatives, cold to the head, mercury, blisters, figure conspicuously, and the cases are supposed to be quite exceptional in which such measures are not required, but it is difficult to assent to all that is taught and practised on this subject.

There are no doubt cases of congestion of the brain and apoplexy, in which the state of coma is unusually prolonged, in which the occurrence of epileptiform convulsion has left the veins of the head and neck in a state of great engorgement, and where it would seem to be the rational course to open a vein and let blood. The danger of apoplexy, or of renewed hæmorrhage, or the engorged state of the lungs, may indeed seem to necessitate such a course. At the same time, much may be done by the application of cold to the head, and by other measures, which will be considered presently; and it certainly may be a question whether bloodletting has any peculiar advantages over those measures. Nay, it may even be a question, whether bloodletting has any advantages at all. No doubt, there is enough of authority in favour of the lancet, but is there enough of reason? Is the theory sound? Is the practice sufficiently encouraging? These are questions which will be answered differently by different persons, and while many will answer unhesitatingly in the affirmative, others will have doubts, which will be expressed in acts, if not in words. If asked, indeed, they may perhaps deny the existence of their doubts, or speak as if they had none; but, in actual practice, the lancet will scarcely be taken out of its case. A great change, indeed, has already taken place, and what the end will be it is difficult to say. In the mean time it would seem to be better to err on the side of doing too little, than on that of doing too much; and on this account, for my own part, I have always dispensed with the lancet, or any mode of bloodletting in cases of congestion of the brain or apoplexy. I have done this without what may seem to be good reason; indeed, I should find it difficult to cite any reason, unless such may be found in the change which has come over the habits of society and the doctrines of the schools. The habits of society are far more temperate than they were formerly, and the people, in consequence, would seem to have become less plethoric and less tolerant of bloodletting. At any rate, plethora is not a common characteristic of patients now-a-days. The doctrines of the schools are also changed or changing in one most important particular. Formerly, every disease was referred to inflammation, and the pathologist was unhappy if he did not discover the traces of this lesion after death; now, many diseases are referred to a process which is the very reverse of inflammation—degeneration, and, instead of bleeding, it has been found to be desirable to enrich the blood and promote nutrition. Nay, the idea of inflammation itself would seem to be undergoing a change, by which it is becoming less fiery or inflammatory, and more akin to the process which has just been named. At any rate, I have not been able to bring my mind to order bleeding in any of these cases; and so far as I am able to form an opinion upon the practice which has fallen to my share up to this time, I have never had occasion to suppose that a better result would have been brought about by a different line of practice.

It is, no doubt, of extreme importance to prevent the accumulation of effete matters in the bowels, and to remove such accumulation when it has taken place, but whether purgatives are the proper remedies is not quite so certain. If the bowels do not act with sufficient regularity there is, in all probability, some error in the diet—some excess of animal food, and some deficiency of culinary vegetables and fruit—and the first thing to be done is, obviously, to correct this error. And this is often all that is wanted, if care be taken to explain to the patient that his bowels can act without purgatives, and that he need not—particularly if advanced or advancing in life—be altogether cast down if now and then they do not act every day. Indeed, if his diet be properly regulated, and this explanation made, the patient will generally have the satisfaction of finding his tongue clean—when he remembers to look at it, and of forgetting his stomach and bowels altogether. Or if the result be not quite so satisfactory, an occasional enema of water or brine upon getting up in the morning will rarely fail to set matters right, and that without disturbing the digestion in any way, or producing any feelings of depression or irritability. There are indeed times in every case where congestion of the brain or apoplexy is a danger to be apprehended, and these times will occur not unfrequently in those cases where the venous system is overloaded and the constitution thoroughly debilitated, where something else may be wanted, where nothing would seem to afford such immediate relief as mercury, and where the *modus operandi* of the medicine, in part at least, would seem to be that of a purgative. In order to produce this relief, however, it is by no means necessary to give the mercury in a quantity sufficient to cause it to act powerfully upon the bowels, or to follow it up by a black draught or other purge, and therefore the good results of this practice cannot be cited as an argument in favour of purging. On the contrary, it would often seem to do most good when it provokes the liver *and kidney* to a natural degree of action. Indeed, I have seen several cases in which the increased action of the kidneys would seem to have had a much greater share in relieving a congested state of the venous system than any increased action of the liver. In cases where the evil has gone further, and the patient has actually been struck down by coma, it may be necessary not only to resort to purgative enemas, but to purge by putting croton oil upon the tongue, or in other

15 §

ways; but even here it can scarcely be said that violent purging is called for.

It is somewhat surprising that *diuretics* have not had a more extensive trial in cases of threatened coma from congestion of the brain, for it might be supposed that remedies of this class would have the power of reducing the quantity of the blood with little or no inconvenience. Indeed, it is only possible to account for this apparent omission by the fact that diuretics are less certain in their action than purgatives. It is not mere theory, however, which would point to diuretics under these circumstances. On the contrary, it has long been the practice of my friend and late colleague, Dr. Hamilton Roe, to give tincture of cantharides in cases of threatened congestion of the brain, with a view to lessening the amount of circulating fluid and relieving the congested veins, by rousing the torpid kidney to a freer action; and in a few cases in which I have had an opportunity of trying this plan of treatment upon my own responsibility, I am able to corroborate the favourable opinion entertained by Dr. Roe. The plan is to give fifteen minims of the tincture in a little mucilage every hour for three or four doses, and the usual result is free secretion of urine and unmistakeable relief to the state of venous congestion, without any of the feelings of depression which so commonly arise from the free action of purgatives. It is not improbable, also, that the quality of the blood may be changed for the better by this freer action of the kidney, for it may be supposed that the increased secretion of urine involves a freer elimination of matters which cause great depression and prostration when retained in the blood—urea and products allied to urea. Where the symptoms of threatened coma are less urgent, colchicum may, perhaps, prove to be a more suitable remedy than cantharides. At any rate, I have often seen the kidney excited to freer action, with unmistakeable relief to the state of venous engorgement, by giving for two or three days a few doses of this tincture, generally in association with sweet spirits of nitre, or by giving a pill containing two grains of the extract of colchicum and one grain of blue pill for two or three nights successively.

Of the importance of applying *cold to the head* there can be no doubt; indeed, this measure may be said to be the natural mode of affording relief in cases of congestion of the brain. If the head be raised, and a stream of cold water poured upon it, particularly if warmth be applied to the feet at the same time, it is indeed difficult to imagine a state of coma which will not yield; and if cold be applied judiciously afterwards, it is as difficult to believe that the coma will not continue in abeyance. At any rate, a state of coma which is manageable in any way may be managed in this way. It would seem, also, that the great difficulty which has always prevented the full realization in practice of the theoretical advantages of cold to the head—the difficulty of applying it for a sufficient length of time, with steadiness, without wetting the patient, and without requiring the whole attention of the nurse—has been overcome by a plan recently proposed by Dr. James Arnott—a plan which for the first time promises to make cold a manageable and available agent in the treatment of disease. "A current of water of the appropriate temperature is made to flow through a thin waterproof cushion in close contact with the body. The water runs into the cushion from a fountain reservoir raised above it, through a long flexible tube; and again, escaping from the cushion, it passes through another tube into the waste vessel. The cushion is of a size and form adapted to the part of the body in which the water is to act; and, by a particular contrivance, any pressure from its weight may be prevented. The part in contact with the cushion is kept moist, either by previously wetting the cushion or by interposing a piece of wet lint, flannel, or other bibulous substance." Speaking of this apparatus, Dr. Watson says that it promises to be an essential auxiliary to the lancet and cupping;

but this, I take it, is not all that may be said. I take it, indeed, that this apparatus will be an essential agent in the treatment of all affections of the head where active inflammation has to be subdued, or where congested veins have to be unloaded, and that it will be a source of great comfort where the sole object is to dispel a feeling of weight or discomfort in the head. I can, indeed, imagine a time when a modification of this apparatus, within the reach of all, may enable any aching and wearied head to enjoy the luxury of a douche or wet towel without the inconvenience of wetting the hair or deranging the dress.

It is not possible that the body or mind can be exerted beyond moderate bounds, or the appetites indulged with impunity where there is a predisposition to congestion of the brain. At the same time it is very possible to err on the side of abstinence, and the necessity for putting the patient on very short commons may well be called in question. It is very desirable to keep down the quantity of the blood, and in order to this it will be of prime importance (seeing that there is often an inactive condition of the kidney) to stint the quantity of sloppy drinks; but it can scarcely be desirable to run the risk of impoverishing the blood, if, as the researches of MM. Andral and Gavaral would seem to show, there is actually less fibrin in the blood of apoplectic patients than there ought to be. In a word, the history of congestion of the brain would not seem to furnish a sound warrant for carrying out what is usually known as the antiphlogistic plan of treatment.

— It would seem, also, that a somewhat similar line of remark is applicable to the treatment of *inflammation of the brain.*

There are cases of inflammation of the brain in which bloodletting may seem to be called for by the intensity of the febrile and inflammatory symptoms; but even in these cases it is difficult to carry out this plan of treatment without some misgiving. For if, as Dr. Bennett maintains,[1] the inflammation in which bloodletting was thought to be most indispensable—inflammation of the lungs, may be treated satisfactorily without bloodletting, may it not be so also with inflammation of the brain? Now it appears, from the investigations of Dr. Bennett, that the result of the rigorous antiphlogistic treatment of pneumonia, as practised formerly in the Edinburgh Infirmary, the Hôpital la Charité at Paris, and in several other hospitals, is a mortality of 1 in 3; that the result of the treatment by tartar emetic in large doses, as practised by Rasori, and more recently by Dietl, is a mortality of 1 in 5, or, according to Laennec, of 1 in 10; that the

'Edinb. Medical Journal,' March, May, June, 1857.

result of moderate bleedings, as in the practice of Grisolle, is a mortality of 1 in 6·50; that the result of a dietetic treatment, with occasional bleedings and emetics in severe cases, as carried out by Skoda, is a mortality of 1 in 7, or, if purely dietetic, as under Dietl, of 1 in 13. It appears, also, that the mortality from pneumonia in the British army, where the malady for the most part has arisen in healthy ablebodied men, is also 1 in 13. And, lastly, it appears that the mortality has been reduced to 1 in 21—to one-seventh, that is to say, of the mortality of twenty years ago—under the treatment pursued by Professor Bennett, during the last eight years, in the Royal Infirmary of Edinburgh. In this practice, no attempt is made to cut the disease short or to weaken the pulse and vital powers, and the sole aim is to facilitate the necessary changes which must take place in the inflammatory exudation before it can be excreted from the system. To this end salines are given in small doses during the period of febrile excitement, and, as soon as the pulse becomes soft, these are changed for good beef-tea and other nutriments. When there is evident weakness, from four to six ounces of wine are allowed daily; and as soon as the period of crisis approaches, the excretion of urates is favoured by giving, three or four times a day, a diuretic, consisting generally of half a drachm of nitric ether, with a few minims of colchicum wine. Or if the crisis occurs by sweating or purging, care is taken not to check it in any way. The question, no doubt, is one of considerable difficulty, and much remains to be proved before an unchallenged answer can be hoped for; but this much is plain, that bleeding and other severe antiphlogistic measures have not been shown to be less necessary now than formerly because inflammation has assumed a more asthenic character, and that authority, however high, must be disallowed, if in such a matter it does not rest upon something more stable than mere precedent. And, if the necessity for bleeding may be called in question in inflammation of the lungs, where the diminution in the respiratory capacity of the lungs would seem to demand a corresponding diminution in the amount of the circulating fluid, it may well be doubted whether bleeding can be regarded as an essential measure in inflammation of the brain. In an organ so delicate as the brain, it is, no doubt, of the highest moment to check inflammatory action as soon as possible; but it is no less important to preserve those reparative powers by which the mischief is to be repaired subsequently, and this the more, seeing that a scrofulous taint may often be detected in inflammation of the brain, and that this inflammation under any circumstances is more akin to degeneration than inflammation elsewhere.

Nor is it easy to assent to the routine practice respecting purgatives. In many cases of inflammation of the brain, the best results will follow the use of purgative enemas at the commencement of the affection, and it will be well to persevere in their use until all effete matters are brought away; but the beneficial results of swallowing purgatives from the beginning to the end are not quite so certain. At any rate, an experience extending over several cases has served to show that there is less sickness where the purgatives are withheld, except in the form of occasional enemas, and that, to say the least, the progress of the case is not less satisfactory.

There are, no doubt, many difficult points to be attended to in the treatment of inflammation of the brain, but much may be done with cold to the head, with a little clear ice, with mercury, with colchicum, with chloroform, if care be taken to keep the sick-room dark and quiet, and the patient himself in a semi-erect posture. Cold to the head is an all important measure, and if much could be done by means of wet rags and bladders containing ice, we may fairly expect that more will be done by means of the apparatus of Dr. James Arnott, already referred to. Applied in this manner, indeed, we may even expect to use cold so as to vanquish any amount of inflammatory action. A little clear ice is also of great service to allay the sickness and quench the thirst. Indeed, a morsel of ice, sucked now and then, will answer these indications better than any kind of effervescing draughts. While the symptoms are at all active, mercury, in all probability, is indispensable, and the most convenient form of giving it will be that of a pill. Two or three grains of calomel in a little conserve, by themselves, or associated with a small quantity of extract of colchicum, and repeated every four hours, may indeed be all the medicine wanted. It is useless, perhaps hurtful, to want to go too fast, and more than enough has been given if the mercury salivate the patient or act violently upon the bowels. By these means, if care be taken to keep the head high, and the sick-room dark and quiet, it is not likely that the inflammation can hold its ground long. Nor is it likely that the pain or delirium should refuse to yield, but if this is not the case, a few whiffs of chloroform will generally be all that is necessary.

The difficulty, however, is not in mastering the inflammation; it is in knowing when to have recourse to restoratives. The question is—are these measures only to be tried, and then very cautiously, as is recommended on high authority—" when an extreme degree of collapse occurs?" Surely not. Surely no theoretical considerations respecting inflammation can justify a plan of treatment which will allow the very faintest degree of collapse to show itself, without at once taking steps to supply food and other restoratives? Surely it cannot be in accordance with any sound rules of physiology or pathology to persevere with antiphlogistic measures until it is dangerous to go on with them any longer, and then at once and suddenly to have recourse to ammonia, Hoffmann's anodyne, beef-tea, wine, and so on?

— If a rigid antiphlogistic plan of treatment is not necessary in inflammation of the brain, it is not likely to be necessary in fever. But, be the treatment of the earlier stage of fever what it may, there can be no doubt that an energetic restorative and stimulant plan of treatment has become necessary when the occurrence of subsultus shows that convulsion is not an unlikely danger.

— Where convulsion has resulted from a suppressed state of the renal and biliary secretions, the patient, in all probability, is sunk in a state of collapse from which there is scarcely any possibility of rousing him, and the local disease, of which the suppression is a sign, is altogether beyond the reach of art; and, therefore, it is of little moment what is done.

— In convulsion depending upon "irritation" in the gums or alimentary canal, the cue as to treatment will have to be taken from the degree of fever and the condition of the circulation in the brain. If there is anything like inflammation in the brain, the remarks which have been already made on this subject are applicable; and the existence of any special cause of irritation, in pointing out an additional cause of exhaustion, would only offer an additional objection to bleeding and purging. Cold to the head, repeated warm-baths, a dose or two of grey powder, lancing the gums or removing any carious teeth, if this be necessary, giving turpentine enemas if worms or effete matters have to be brought away, with beef-tea from the beginning, and wine and other restoratives very soon after the beginning,—such are the measures which would seem to be necessary. Where convulsion is connected with irritation in the uterus, or in the sexual apparatus, some special local measures may be required; but there is no reason for supposing that the general treatment will be different from that which has been pointed out when speaking of epileptic and hysteric convulsion, except in this— that the very presence of the "irritation" would seem to be an additional reason for distrusting any measures of a lowering character. Where convulsion arises in connexion with puerperal fever, the circumstances are for the most part analogous to those belonging to the convulsion connected with ordinary fever, and the treatment also must be analogous. With respect to the convulsion of flooding, only one course can be proper, and that is to keep the patient alive by wine, transfusion of blood, and so on. Indeed, there is only one case under the present head in which the history of the convulsion would seem to demand a different treatment to that which has appeared to be necessary up to this point, and this is the convulsion occurring in labour without flooding. Now, in this case, the head is often greatly congested, and the aëration of the blood is seriously interfered with, partly as a consequence of the way in which the lungs sympathise with the suffering brain, and partly because the regular movements of the chest are greatly interfered with by the constant straining. Now, if bleeding can be necessary in any case, it must be in this, for these constant strainings are continually putting the patient in danger of fresh convulsion and apoplexy, by the way in which they interfere with the respiratory movements and prevent the free return of blood from the brain. At the same time, it may be well even here to procure a state of artificial rest by means of chloroform vapour, and to take some steps for relieving the uterus of its burden, before having recourse to this measure.

— And, lastly, it is scarcely to be supposed that there is anything in the history of the epileptiform convulsion connected with the moribund state which can invalidate the conclusion which arises uniformly out of all the previous considerations.

CHAPTER V.

OF SPASM.

THE third category of convulsive diseases is characterised by prolonged muscular contraction or spasm. It includes catalepsy, tetanus, cholera, hydrophobia, ergotism, the rigidity of cerebral paralysis, the spasm connected with certain diseases of the spinal cord, and other spasms of a minor character.

The history of spasm.

1. In *catalepsy* the muscles become rigid and slightly contracted, and the patient retains the expression of countenance and the posture which he had before the seizure. The muscles also are pliable, and if the position of the limbs be altered it is retained. The appearance during the attack is that of a corpse, and the condition is only one short degree removed from that of a corpse. In some instances, however, the muscular rigidity is less marked, the corpse-like sleep less profound, the pulse less imperceptible, the face and head less pale and cool than the rest of the body; and, in other instances, there may be less activity in the respiration

than in the circulation, and, as a consequence of this, the veins of the head and neck may stand out somewhat more distinctly; but usually the state is one which may easily be mistaken for that of a corpse.

2. The spasms of *tetanus* begin in the muscles of the face, and give to the features a drawn and aged expression; they then lay hold upon the muscles of the neck, jaws, and throat, and, lastly, they extend to the limbs, to the trunk, and even to the interior of the body. In the height of the disorder the eyeballs may be firmly fixed, and the tongue stiff and immoveable. Sometimes all muscles are affected equally; sometimes certain groups are affected more than others, in which case the jaws may be locked and the rest of the body free, or the body may be bent backwards, forwards, or sideways, as the case may be. The spasms occur in paroxysms, without any perfect remissions, except during sleep. At first the surface of the body is of the natural heat and colour, but as the malady progresses the temperature falls and the skin becomes drenched in perspiration. The respiration, never free, becomes more and more laboured as the spasm gripes with firmer hold upon the respiratory muscles, and towards the end there are moments in which the struggle for breath is agonizing. The pulse, never excited by the least semblance of fever,

soon becomes feeble and frequent, except during the moments of unusual difficulty of breathing, and then the colour of the skin shows very clearly that any increase of fulness, if such there be, is not altogether due to the injection of red blood into the arteries. The reflex excitability of the system is greatly increased, and ordinary impressions on the senses are sufficient to bring on a paroxysm. As to the rest, there is, with very few exceptions, excruciating pain in the cramped parts, at the pit of the stomach, and in the wound or cicatrix, if such there be; and, lastly, there is no stupor, except towards the end, when the action of the brain has begun to suffer from the circulation of imperfectly aërated blood. The causes of this sad malady are not at all obvious. Wounds, no doubt, are a most important cause, and in some instances these would seem to have acted by depriving the patient of blood, by the shock to the system, or by the natural depression resulting from the thoughts of danger or of a maimed and helpless future; but in other instances the history of the case presents nothing so obvious, and it is necessary to be content with the supposition that the wound has set up a state of inflammation or "irritation" in a nerve, and that the propagation of this state to the nervous centres is the cause of all the evil. Wounds, however, are not necessary to the production of tetanus, and wounds, in all probability, are never of themselves sufficient. At any rate, it is the opinion of army surgeons that tetanus is most apt to occur when soldiers are dispirited, exhausted, ill-fed, and exposed to cold.

With respect to the appearances after death, some very valuable information is presented in a recent report, by Mr. Poland, of 72 cases of tetanus which occurred in Guy's Hospital between 1825 and 1857.[1] Thus, of 20 cases in which the *brain* was examined, this organ was found to be healthy in 11, congested in 4, darker than natural in 1, dark and flabby in 1, pinkish in 1, ulcerated on the under surface of the anterior lobes in 1 (the result of injury to the head co-existing with the tetanus), decomposed in 1 (an acute case, fatal in four days, the examination being made forty-one hours after death, and the muscles still remaining rigid). Of 19 cases in which the spinal cord was examined, this organ was healthy in 8, firm, rigid, and of pinkish hue in 1, of natural firmness but injected in 1, congested in 2, darker than natural in 1, pinkish in 2, of a "higher tint" in 1, softened in 1, decomposed in 1 (the case in which the brain was decomposed). Of 14 cases in which the nerve at the seat of the wound was examined, the nerve was healthy in 3, inflamed in 5, a divided nerve

[1] 'Guy's Hospital Reports,' 3d series, vol. iii, 1857.

united in 2, the end bulbous in 1, the nervous twigs entering the cicatrix pinkish in 1, and of the remaining 2 the filaments of the facial nerve were spread over the ulcer, but their condition not stated in 1, and in the other, in which tetanus followed amputation through the thigh, the divided sciatic nerve lay exposed to the extent of two inches, with granulations around and over it, but the nerve itself apparently healthy. Of the appearances in other organs nothing need be said.

3. The cramps of *cholera* begin in the alimentary canal, and extend successively to the abdomen, thighs, legs, chest, arms, and hands, and, once established, they continue, with few intermissions, until death. The surface of the body is cold, clammy, and blue. The pulse rapidly becomes insensible. The respiration is laboured and panting, and the breath cold. The sense of pain and suffering is greatly blunted, for the mental energies have succumbed to the blow which has prostrated the bodily powers.

4. The spasms of *hydrophobia* occur in paroxysms, which increase in violence and recur more frequently as the malady progresses. They begin in suffocative and strangulatory contractions of the muscles concerned in respiration and deglutition; then they extend to the limbs and trunk; and, eventually, they may seize upon the bladder and intestines.

In some instances, the disorder has been mistaken for tetanus. In the intervals there is the greatest inquietude and restlessness, and every voluntary movement is hurried, impulsive, almost convulsive. Occasionally, there is unceasing tremor and tremulous agitation. The hands and feet are cool and cold, and so is the surface generally, though in a less marked degree. The pulse is quick and feeble, and the respiration quickened and often interrupted by sobs and sighs. The mental state is one of fear or even despair, with occasional outbursts of delirious violence, in which there is a tendency to injure, sometimes to bite, others. There is more or less pain in the wound or cicatrix, and—what is far more distressing than any mere pain—there is a distressing sense of suffocation as from some impediment in the throat. The most marked and distressing symptom, however, is the excessive irritability of the whole system, and the extreme facility with which a paroxysm may be brought on by the most insignificant cause. A gust of air, a beam of light, a sudden noise, a single touch, may be sufficient for the purpose. The gullet is not less sensitive, and because drinking, or any attempt to drink, provokes the paroxysm, the patient dreads to drink, though he does not fear the water, as the name of the disease would imply. All the secretions appear natural, except the saliva, which is viscid and abundant. This secretion is a source of great distress to the patient, for it cannot be swallowed or expectorated without great difficulty, nor can it be rinsed away, for the contact of water with the throat brings on the paroxysm.

The appearances after death in 46 cases, the histories of which were carefully analysed by my brother,[1] teach us that " the disease may be fully developed, run its course, and terminate fatally, without leaving any appreciable lesion of structure, that the lesions which are observed in certain cases are not constant," . . . . " that no satisfactory link of connexion can be found in many, if in any, instances, between the appearances observed after death and the symptoms noted during life." . . . . " In the majority of cases, however, there were indications, more or less marked, of morbid action in various organs. Thus, morbid appearances were found in the dura mater in 8 cases, in the arachnoid in 10, in the pia mater in 16, in the velum interpositum in 2, in the choroid plexus in 12, in the cerebral hemispheres in 28, in the spinal cord and membranes in 18, in the medulla oblongata and pons varolii in 4, in the cerebro-spinal and sympathetic nerves in 4, in the tongue in 8, in the palate in 3, in the salivary glands in 2, in the pharynx in 19, in the œsophagus in 16, in the stomach in

'Lancet,' September, 1856.

20, in the intestines in 6, in the larynx, trachea, and bronchial tubes in 31, in the ultimate ramifications of the air-passages in 24, in the heart in 4. These lesions consisted of every grade of injection of the blood-vessels, from the slightest blush to the most vivid, or dark, black congestion; of alterations in the consistency of the tissues, principally softening; effusion of blood, and certain products of perverted nutrition and secretion. In several of the cases the lesions were of such a character that they have been classed with those resulting from common idiopathic inflammation; in a greater number of cases the lesions were of that character which is found in structural changes occurring in asthenic conditions of the system."

5. The cramps of *ergotism*, according to Romberg, who borrows his description from the accounts supplied by Wichmann, Taube and Wagner, occur in the following manner—" The feet and hands are attacked with cramp in the flexor muscles. The fingers of both hands are bent like hooks, the thumb being pushed under the fore and middle fingers in an oblique direction, the wrist is strongly curved inwards, so that the hand assumes the shape of an eagle's beak. The toes are also doubled under the foot. The spasm extends over the fore and upper arm, which are bent one upon another at an acute angle; it also extends over the thigh and legs, and

over the back of the neck and jaws." These symptoms end either in tetanus or epileptiform convulsion. The skin is dull and dry, except during the paroxysm, when it is perspiring. The pulse and respiration are affected in the same way as in tetanus. All the senses are considerably dulled, and that of feeling is well-nigh annihilated. The cramps are accompanied with pain, which is generally relieved by extending the cramped parts. At first, the intelligence is not sensibly affected, but it fails as the disease proceeds, and before death the state may be almost one of fatuity. As the disease proceeds, also, paralysis may supplant the cramps. If life is prolonged sufficiently, a state of slow mortification is set up in the extremities, and the fingers and toes, or even the hands and feet, may have disappeared before death. The main cause of this malady is the habitual use of grain affected with the ergot disease, and a residence in the low, malarious, damp districts in which this disease takes its origin.

6. The *rigidity of cerebral paralysis* may come on at the moment of the cerebral attack or shortly afterwards, or it may be deferred for a while; and this difference in the time of occurrence, as Dr. Todd has very well pointed out, is a very important difference.

(*a.*) In the " early rigidity," or that which comes on at the moment of the attack or shortly afterwards, Dr. Todd indicates two varieties—one in which the rigidity is slight and confined to one or two muscles, the other in which the state is co-extensive with the paralysis. Where the rigidity is slight and partial, it may only appear when the muscles are put on the stretch. In this way, the biceps may become stiff and rigid, and prevent perfect extension of the arm, or the triceps may contract in the same manner and prevent perfect flexion of the arm, or a similar affection of the flexores digitorum may make it impossible to stretch out the fingers to the full. This rigidity is more commonly manifested in the flexor muscles than in the extensors, and most of all in the flexors of the arms and hands : it is rarely met with in the muscles of the face. In its most marked degree it is firm and constant. In these cases, the nutrition of the muscles is not materially damaged at first, and there is little or no wasting ; but after a while, if the palsy continue, the muscles waste away, though never so rapidly as in those cases of paralysis in which the muscles are loose and flabby from the beginning. At first, also, the circulation in the part is vigorous, the heat is maintained at the proper standard, and the muscles are as sensitive to the galvanic current as they were before the paralysis, or even more sensitive.

(b) " Late rigidity," or that form which does

not occur for some time after the paralysis, may seize upon those muscles which were left by the paralysis in a lax and flabby state, or it may supervene, with or without any interval, upon "early rigidity." It never happens until the paralysed muscles have wasted considerably; it is established by slow degrees; and where it is perfect, the wasted muscles are stretched like tense cords between their points of attachment. It agrees with "early rigidity" in its preference for the flexor muscles, particularly for the flexors of the upper extremity, and when it is most marked in this latter part, the forearm may be tightly flexed upon the upper arm, and the fingers as tightly bent into the palm. In this form of rigidity the muscles are always wasted, and they may be reduced to mere membranous shreds. And as might be expected from this state of wasting, the circulation in the paralysed parts is very feeble, and the heat very imperfectly maintained. It would seem, also, that the muscles have ceased to respond to the influence of galvanism before they pass into this state of rigidity. At any rate they do not respond to this influence after they have passed into this state.

7. The spinal cord is subject to all the diseases which may affect the brain, and spasm may be a symptom in almost any case; but it is only necessary here to trace the history of *spasm as. connected*

with active disease of the spinal cord—inflammation and apoplexy.

(*a.*) The symptoms of *acute spinal meningitis* are pain in the neighbourhood of the affected part, violent from the beginning and rapidly becoming almost intolerable, increased by motion, and by the application of a hot sponge, but not by pressure—pains and feelings of pricking or numbness in the course of the nerves proceeding from the affected part, and a cord-like sense of constriction around the body upon a level with this part—spasms in the muscles of the back and neck, increased by motion and varying in severity from mere stiffness to complete opisthotonos—often increased susceptibility in the sense of touch—spasmodic breathing—obstinate constipation—retention of urine—and if the inflamed part be higher than the lumbar region of the cord—priapism. "The cramp," says Dr. Romberg, "is rarely persistent, being generally remittent, and recurring spontaneously after a pause, or as soon as the patient is required to make a movement." The lower limbs, and the upper limbs too if the mischief be sufficiently high, are feeble, but not paralysed. At first, the mind is little affected, but as the disease progresses, a state of coma, sometimes preceded by wild delirium, may be developed. At first, there may be symptoms of active fever, but if so, these very rapidly lapse into those belonging to the typhoid condition. Indeed, in all cases the powers of the system must soon succumb to want of air, for the respiration is difficult and laboured from the beginning. Acute spinal meningitis is not unfrequently associated with the corresponding disease of the brain, and among the assigned causes, local violence, exposure to cold, and great fatigue, take the highest rank. Spinal meningitis in a chronic form is rarely met with, except in connexion with caries of the vertebræ, and its symptoms are for the most part sufficiently obvious— paroxysms of pain in the neighbourhood of the part affected and along the nerves connected with this part, paralysis of motion extending centripetally, stiffness and spasm in the muscles of the neck and back, hectic, emaciation, œdema of the legs, a peculiarly dry and scurfy condition of the skin, and before death mischief in the brain of one kind or another.

Myelitis, however rapid in its course, has few of the characteristics of an acute disease. Its symptoms are feelings of numbness and tingling or pain beginning in the fingers and toes and creeping upwards, a sensation as of a cord tied around the body upon the level of the affected part, and paralysis of the regions below this part. Pain in the back is not a prominent symptom, and what little there is, though increased by heat, is not materially aggravated by motion—a point in which this pain differs essentially from that of acute spinal meningitis; but pains in the parts to which the nerves connected with the diseased spine are distributed, often of considerable severity, are not at all uncommon. The characteristic symptom, indeed, is paralysis, not spasm or pain, and in some instances there may be scarcely any pain or spasm from the beginning to the end of the malady. If the site of the disease be low down, the paralysis may be confined to the legs, and life may be prolonged for a considerable time; if the site be sufficiently high, all parts of the body may be paralysed except the head, and death may be speedily brought about by paralysis of the muscles connected with the processes of respiration and deglutition. In the beginning the mind is clear, but this clearness is of short duration, and eventually the state is one of coma. The circulation never exhibits the slightest tendency to excitement. On the contrary, there is almost from the beginning a marked disposition to mortification in all parts which have to bear anything like pressure—a disposition which is utterly inconsistent with anything like true activity in the circulation. The symptoms of chronic myelitis, which most frequently make their appearance in connexion with caries of the vertebræ, would seem to differ from those which have just been mentioned in nothing beyond the comparative slowness of their development. They are always accompanied by hectic disturbance and extreme emaciation.

(*b.*) The immediate symptoms of *spinal apoplexy* are pain and marked paralysis of motion. If the site of the hæmorrhage be sufficiently high, there will be great dyspnœa and convulsive agitation and spasm in the parts below the injury. If the site be still higher, death may happen at once. If life be prolonged, there is rapid wasting, and a great tendency to slough away in all parts below the injured portion of the cord.

8. Every muscle, or group of muscles, in the body, may be affected with spasm, and it is necessary to glance at a few of the more important of these *minor forms of spasm*.

A patient may squint in various ways from a spasmodic state of one or other of the muscles of the eye, and this state may be brought about in various ways. It may be symptomatic of acute or chronic disease of the brain, particularly of the base of this organ; it may have been set up by the irritation of teething or worms; it may have been caused by the habit of turning the eye so as to keep some opaque portion of the cornea out of the line of vision; or it may have been brought about in several other ways.

The muscles of the face and tongue may be affected in various degrees with spasm, and a very common cause of the limitation of the spasm to these particular muscles will be found to be some irritation proceeding from the teeth. In some of these cases, the way in which the spasm ceases when the cause of irritation is removed is not a little remarkable. A case in point is related by Mr. Mitchell, in the fourth volume of the 'Medico-Chirurgical Transactions,' and quoted by Dr. Romberg:

CASE.—"A female, æt. 50, was suddenly attacked with spasms of the facial muscles and tongue, which, after the lapse of a fortnight, extended to the neck. The paroxysm commenced with a sense of weakness and oppression at the præcordia, and a violent shooting pain passing from the sternum to the spine, rising upwards to the tongue, which then became as stiff as a piece of wood, bending the point upwards to the left side of the arch of the palate. A sense of numbness attacked the left side of the nose and the chin. The left angle of the mouth was opened and distorted, the teeth were closely compressed, all the muscles of the face became rigidly contracted, the nose was drawn over to the left side, and the forehead and eyebrows were corrugated by the spasm of the occipito-frontal and corrugator supercilii muscles. The muscles of the neck rotated the head to the left shoulder, the left arm became extended, and a sense of numbness ran down in a straight line from the neck to the thumb and forefinger. Consciousness and the action of heart and lungs continued unaffected. After three minutes there was a remission, commencing with a tremor of all the affected muscles. These paroxysms returned day and night at intervals of ten minutes. As the treatment pursued produced no effect, another physician was consulted, who had seen a similar case of facial and lingual spasm cured by the extraction of a carious tooth; on examining the teeth of this patient, though she did not complain of toothache, one tooth was found in the upper left row to be in a morbid condition and sensitive to the touch. The gum was inflamed and a fetid matter discharged. After the first molar was extracted and the gums had been scarified, the paroxysms diminished in intensity and frequency, and they entirely ceased after the extraction of all the carious teeth."

In some of these cases the spasm is accompanied by tic-douloureux, and the spasm and pain may be relieved at one and the same time by the removal of the source of irritation.

The jaw may also be locked by the spasm of some of the muscles concerned in mastication, or the head may be pulled down or twisted awry by a corresponding spasm in the muscles of the neck; and these symptoms may point to mischief in the brain or upper part of the spinal chord, as well as to the ordinary sources of irritation.

"Writer's cramp," again, is a local spasmodic affection of the muscles of the hand and arm. In this affection, every attempt to write produces spasm in the muscles of the thumb and two adjoining fingers, and sometimes in those of the forearm and upper arm, and, what is not a little curious, these very muscles are capable of performing every other movement but those which are involved in the act of writing. An analogous kind of cramp may also be provoked by an attempt to perform other acts. Thus: Dr. Romberg speaks of a blacksmith, whose right arm became rigid and painful whenever he took hold of the hammer and attempted to strike. In all these cases, local exhaustion from inordinate exertion of the affected muscles would seem to be the main cause of the trouble

Spasmodic contraction of the hip-joint or clubfoot are the principal forms in which spasm affects the inferior extremities. In some of these cases the spasms are only brought on by a particular mode of exercising the muscles. Dr. Romberg cites three cases in point—cases of periodic clubfoot—from the works of Stromeyer and Dieffenbach, and of these the following is one :[1]

CASE.—" Mr. Von J—, æt. 22, a student of philosophy, robust and in florid health, was attacked in his early youth with a debility of the lower extremities, rendering locomotion difficult. The examination of the extremities showed no difference either in form or nutrition. In the sitting posture both feet were perfectly well formed, and the young man was able to make every movement with facility; but if he rose and walked, his gait was insecure, tottering, and waddling, resembling the movements of a person upon polished ice with smooth boots. His walk became more irregular when he took off his boots and

[1] Op. cit., vol. i, p. 325.

stockings, and walked barefoot through the room; he was then often obliged to support himself to prevent his falling. If he placed his feet on the ground, their form was normal; but as soon as he rose from his chair, and the feet had to bear the weight of the body, they instantly assumed the shape of splay feet, the arch of the sole disappeared, the toes contracted and were raised with the front of the foot, so that the dorsum of the foot presented a concavity."

The hands and feet may also be the seat of other spasmodic affections, and the contractions called "carpopedal convulsions" are an instance in point. These spasms may occur periodically and remain for days and weeks at a time. They flex the thumb across the palm and bend the fingers over it; sometimes they bend the entire hand upon the wrist; they double the toes inwardly and extend the foot. These spasms are unattended with pain, but any attempt at extension makes the patient cry out. They are confined to the first three years of life; they are often associated with some other spasmodic affection, as laryngismus stridulus, and, so far as is known, they do not depend upon any special cause.

Cramp in the muscles of the calves is another very common form of minor spasm. It occurs more frequently in women than in men, and most frequently in the more irritable and weakly of women. It is the close companion of tremulousness; it increases in frequency as age advances. It is very prone to happen during sleep, and the liability to it is infinitely increased during a state of fatuity. In this form of spasm the circulation in the limb is always very inactive, and not unfrequently the system is depressed at the time by some bowel complaint—diarrhœa or dysentery, or by pain, as from sciatica.

Or spasm may attack muscles belonging to the involuntary system, particularly the muscles of the larynx, as in laryngismus stridulus and hooping cough.

The spasm of laryngismus stridulus occurs suddenly and without any very obvious premonition. It may be a solitary phenomenon; it may be associated with cramps in the hands and feet, or with general convulsions; or it may alternate with these cramps and convulsions. So long as it lasts, the spasm causes an agony of suffocation. When it is over, the air finds admission to the lungs with a crowing sound, and the patient is relieved. There is no pain, no alteration of voice, no fever, and in these negative features the affection differs mainly from croup.

Nor is the history of the analogous spasm of hooping cough less marked. The disease in which this spasm arises has two stages—the catarrhal and the convulsive. The first of these is attended by all the symptoms of coryza or catarrh, the cough being more sonorous and violent than usual, but *without any hoop.* The second stage is marked by the subsidence of all febrile disturbance, and by the supervention of the hoop. The hoop, moreover, disappears if pneumonia or bronchitis be developed after its establishment, and remains in abeyance so long as the inflammation continues. In the paroxysm itself the general condition is that of suffocation.

Besides these forms of spasm there are several others—in the bronchial muscles, in the walls of the chest and abdomen, causing hiccup, yawning, sneezing, cough, and so on; but these are physiological questions rather than pathological, and (after what has been said already) it is scarcely necessary to enter into them here.

The pathology of spasm.

(*a.*) *The pathology of spasm as deduced from a consideration of the phenomena connected with the vascular system.*

In all varieties of spasm there is no evidence whatever of excitement of the circulation, and such evidence as there is is altogether of a contrary significance.

In catalepsy the appearance during the attack is that of a corpse. The blood is well-nigh stagnant in the vessels, and it may be necessary to apply a stethoscope to the heart to know of a certainty that the patient lives.

In tetanus there is no fever. All observers are agreed upon this point. It is found, also, that the extremities become colder and colder, that the heart beats with greater feebleness as the malady progresses, and that the spasms become more general and more violent as this change takes place. Nor is the congested, warm, and perspiring skin of the body and neck an argument to the contrary, for this state is accounted for, partly by the blood being driven out of the contracted muscles, and partly by that law of compensation by which the blood is diverted to the surface, and the skin made to do duty for the lungs when these organs are impeded in their action. Moreover, the bouts of spasm are distinctly coincident with paroxysms of difficulty of breathing, and in this way the spasm would seem to be connected, not with over-action of the circulation, but with a state in which the aëration of the blood is considerably interfered with. And in the tetanus caused by strychnia there is an additional cause of vascular depression—a cause which may be considered as equivalent to a considerable loss of blood, or to an advanced stage of suffocation—for, as Dr. Harley has pointed out (p. 91), the effect of the poison is to make the blood less stimulating by rendering it less capable of combining with oxygen, and at the same time to diminish, in no inconsiderable degree, the irritability of the muscle.

In the spasms of cholera the skin is frigid and clammy and blue, the breath cold, the pulse well-nigh imperceptible, and that the coincidence of this state of collapse with the spasm is more than accidental would seem to be evident, in the fact that the spasm relaxes *pari passu* with the reaction of recovery.

In hydrophobia the state of the circulation is the very opposite of fever, as is proved by the cold hands and feet, the perspiring skin, the quick and feeble pulse, the sobbing and sighing respiration, as well as by the fact that the agitation and spasm and convulsion increase in violence as the circulation fails. Sometimes, as in a case recently related by Dr. Lawrie, of Glasgow,[1] the pulse is more active. In this case "the pulse was 150, regular, but not strong"—not strong, but evidently stronger than is usual in hydrophobia. But in this case there was also far less convulsive disturbance than usual, and the symptoms were more like those of acute hysteria than anything else. "The globus and incessant tossings were well marked; but although the desire to move was irresistible, the movements had no appearance of being involuntary or associated with insensibility." Cases

[1] 'Edinb. Med. Journal,' August, 1852.

like this, therefore, where the circulation is less depressed than usual, are only calculated to confirm the idea that this very depression is connected with the spasm and convulsion.

In ergotism, so far as we know, the pulse presents no sign of excitement throughout the whole course of the malady.

In the "early rigidity" of cerebral paralysis there is at first no very evident alteration in the circulation, and the heat does not fall below the normal standard, but before long both pulse and heat fail in the paralysed parts. In "late rigidity" the local circulation is always feeble, and the heat in the part is kept up with great difficulty.

In acute spinal meningitis there may be symptoms of active fever at the onset, but if so they very shortly lapse into those belonging to a typhoid condition. Usually, however, the symptoms have a typhoid aspect from the beginning, and the respiration is too laboured and imperfect to allow of a different state of things. In acute myelitis the circulation is utterly without power, and as an additional evidence of this, there is a marked disposition to slough in all parts subjected to pressure. In chronic spinal meningitis and in chronic myelitis, the state is the last degree of hectic exhaustion.

In the different forms of minor spasm there is for the most part no evidence of over-action in the circulation. Nor is it otherwise where the phenomena of fever would seem to be mixed up with the spasm, as in hooping-cough. For what is the fact? The fact is that the hoop, which is the audible sign of the spasm, does not make its appearance until the febrile or catarrhal stage has passed off; that it disappears if pneumonia, bronchitis, or any other inflammation be developed in the course of the malady; and that it returns again when the inflammation has departed. In this case, also, as in laryngismus stridulus, the way in which the spasm is mixed up with the phenomena of partial suffocation is an argument that the spasm is favoured by imperfectly arterialised blood—by a state, that is to say, which involves a corresponding degree of vascular depression.

— In a word, the conclusion arising from a consideration of the phenomena connected with the vascular system, is in harmony with the conclusion already drawn with respect to tremor and convulsion, and the spasm is seen to be connected, not with over-action of the circulation, but with a state which is diametrically opposed to this.

(b.) *The pathology of spasm as deduced from a consideration of the phenomena connected with the nervous system.*

In the more severe forms of the disorders which

are characterised by spasm, the mental state is indicative of exhaustion, prostration, or inaction. In catalepsy the mind is in abeyance, or when otherwise its manifestations are at most an obscure dream. In tetanus the patient is alarmed, absorbed in his sufferings, agitated. The cramps of cholera are attended by indifference to the future and utter hopelessness, than which there are no surer signs of utter mental prostration. In hydrophobia everything denotes the want of mental energy, for the state is not unlike that of delirium tremens. The patient is overcome with dread. In ergotism the mental state before death may be little short of fatuity. In both forms of the rigidity of cerebral paralysis, early as well as late, the brain has been seriously damaged by white-softening, by apoplectic effusion, by red-softening, or in some other way, and the mental power has suffered accordingly. Nor is the case different in other forms of spasm. There may not be such obvious want of mental power, but if a careful search be made, there is always certain evidence of some want.

The state of the mind, indeed, is what might be expected from the depressed state of the circulation, and the depressed state of the circulation (to pursue the argument already used on more than one occasion) is one which necessitates, as it would seem, a corresponding state of inaction, not only in the brain, but in the medulla oblongata, spinal cord, and all other parts of the nervous system. At the same time there are sundry difficulties which must be removed before such a conclusion can be accepted.

There can be no difficulty in accepting this conclusion with respect to catalepsy, for here the corpse-like condition may be fairly referred to a corpse-like deprivation of life, mental and corporeal.

Nor are the traces of inflammation which are occasionally met with in the brain or spinal cord or nerves of persons dying of tetanus, an objection to the idea that there is no over-action of the nervous system during tetanus. It is evident that inflammation of these organs is not an essential condition of the disease, for in the majority of cases, as in the cases dying in Guy's Hospital since 1825, there is not the smallest trace of such a lesion. Nay, it may even be said that the inflammation has served to mitigate or antagonize the tetanic contractions, for it is certain that these contractions may be developed in their most violent and perfect form where inflammation is most unequivocally absent, and that they may be absent where inflammation is as unequivocally present. And, certainly, there is no necessity to call in the aid of any over-action of the nervous system to account for the exalted susceptibility to reflex movement which is so marked a feature of the tetanic state. On the contrary, it has been seen that there is the same exalted susceptibility in cases where the natural supply of nervous influence to the part has been diminished. Thus, it is more easy to provoke reflex movements in the hind legs of a frog after the influence of the brain has been cut off by dividing the cord; and it is more easy still to do this after the influence of the cord as well as the brain has been cut off by dividing the sciatic nerves. It has been seen, also, that the *modus operandi* of strychnia in producing a state which is strictly analogous to ordinary tetanus is one which is altogether opposed to the idea of over-action in the nervous system, for it is found that the nervous as well as the muscular structures are rendered less irritable by the poison, and that the blood is changed in such a way as to make it less capable of exciting the action of the system generally.

In cholera, as in catalepsy, it would seem to be gratuitous to suppose that inflammation or any other process of excitement has anything to do with the phenomena of the cramps.

In hydrophobia, as in tetanus, the symptoms have been referred to inflammation in some portion of the cerebro-spinal axis, and there are many cases in which the traces of such a lesion are unmistakeably present after death. In hydrophobia, however, as in tetanus, there are other cases, scarcely if at all less numerous, in which there are no such traces, and hence it is impossible to suppose that inflammation is essential to the existence of the malady. With respect to the influence of the wound, there would seem to be only one conclusion, and this is one which may perhaps throw some light upon the real nature of the connexion between inflammation and the hydrophobic symptoms. It would seem that the system has been inoculated with a certain virus by the tooth of the rabid animal, and that the effects of this inoculation are fully developed at the time when the symptoms of the disease declare themselves. It would seem, indeed, as if the steps of this history were in some degree parallel with those of smallpox. In smallpox there is a virus. This is introduced by inoculation. For a time the workings within the system are scarcely perceptible. Then rigors and other symptoms of collapse make their appearance, and the system is suddenly laid prostrate. And lastly, there is a period of febrile reaction, in which inflammation and suppuration is set up in the skin and elsewhere. In hydrophobia, also, there is a virus. It has been introduced by inoculation. The baneful workings are hid for a season, and then, suddenly breaking out, the system is overwhelmed by the fearful collapse of the disease. It would seem as if no other hypothesis but that of a poison working in this way upon the blood could account for the suddenness of the outburst, and for the rapidity with which the fatal result is brought about. And if so, then the disease becomes removed in a sense from the category of idiopathic inflammations to that of fevers, and without any great stretch of fancy the evidences of inflammation—suppuration and the rest—are made to take the same position in relation to the fundamental disorder that they do in smallpox. Without any great stretch of fancy, that is to say, the evidences of inflammation in the cerebro-spinal axis and in other parts may be supposed to be as distinctly secondary to the collapse of hydrophobia, as are the corresponding signs of inflammation and suppuration in the skin and elsewhere to the initial period of collapse in smallpox. In other words, the idea of inflammation may be said to change in some degree into that of a depurative, and therefore a curative process, for this is the view which is presented to us by the history of smallpox. According to this view, indeed, the absence of inflammatory appearances would tend to show that death had happened before there had been time for such appearances to be developed, and, to return to the former illustration, the case would be analogous to a one of smallpox in which death had happened in the period of rigor or collapse which precedes the development of the characteristic pustules. And, certainly, it would seem to be an argument in favour of the view here taken, that the traces of inflammation in hydrophobia are met with almost anywhere and everywhere, as they would be if they were secondary, so to speak, to some lesion in the blood. This vagueness in the seat of the inflammation is well seen in my brother's analysis of 46 cases already referred to. And as to the extreme susceptibility to reflex movement which is so marked a feature in hydrophobia, there is no reason for supposing that the explanation is different to that which applied to the corresponding symptom in tetanus.

In ergotism there is no evidence of inflammation or quasi-excitement of any kind to complicate the matter, and from the beginning the system would seem to be poisoned and depressed by the diseased grain, the eating of which has been one main cause the malady.

Nor is it necessary to suppose, with Dr. Todd, that the "early rigidity" of cerebral paralysis is dependent upon a certain irritation which is propagated from the torn portion of the brain to the point into which the nerves of the affected muscles are implanted, and that "late rigidity" is consequent upon the irritation arising from the contraction of the cicatrix by which the cerebral lesion, apoplectic or other, is repaired. For what are the facts? In "early rigidity" the local circulation is vigorous, the heat has not fallen below the natural standard, the muscles are not sensibly wasted, and they promptly respond to the influence of galvanism. The condition of the circulation, that is to say, is favourable to the preservation of the physical and functional integrity, not only of the paralysed muscles, but of the nerves by which these muscles communicate with the brain. In this case, indeed, the muscles are no longer under the control of the will, but they have still some connexion with the brain, for it may be supposed that the nerves are able, in part at least, to discharge their office of conductors. In this case, that is to say, the nerves being conductors, the muscles may still respond to that change in the brain—a loss of action according to the premises—of which contraction is the result. And thus it may be supposed that the contraction of "early rigidity" is brought about, because the portion of the brain connected with the nerves proceeding to the muscles is left permanently in that state in which it is held momentarily during the time that the will is occupied in causing muscular contraction. In "late rigidity," on the contrary, the circulation is very feeble, the heat is very imperfectly maintained, and the muscles are wasted and unable to respond to the influence of galvanism. The condition of the circulation, that is to say, is not favourable to the maintenance of the physical and functional integrity of the paralysed muscles and nerves. The condition of the circulation, in other words, is not favourable to the maintenance of the muscular and nerve-currents, and, becoming less favourable every day, a time at length arrives when these currents die out altogether and allow the muscles to pass into the state of contraction. And thus, according to the premises, it may be supposed that "late rigidity" is nothing more than the anticipation of *rigor mortis*—a *rigor mortis in vitâ*.

There are numerous instances on record of inflammation of the spinal cord or its membranes without any symptoms of a tetanic character, and therefore it is not to be supposed that inflammation is necessarily concerned in the production of spasm in these cases. On the contrary, it is as easy, if not easier, to suppose that the inflammation has antagonised or mitigated the spasm. For if violent and general tetanic symptoms may be developed in cases where the spinal cord is altogether untouched by inflammation, as in many cases of tetanus; and if these tetanic symptoms are comparatively slight and confined to the back and neck, where the spinal cord is actually and unmistakeably inflamed; is it not fair to suppose that the inflammation has had the effect of antagonising or mitigating the spasm?

Nor is it likely that inflammation of the nervous system is more necessary to the production of the minor forms of spasm, for if the help of this state may be dispensed with in the major forms of spasmodic disorder, it is not likely to be required in the explanation of these minor forms.

— As in the different varieties of tremor and convulsion, therefore, so in the different varieties of spasm, the facts are at complete variance with the idea that the muscles are provoked to excessive contraction by excessive stimulation of any kind. The facts, it would seem, are at complete variance with this idea, and in as complete harmony with that doctrine of muscular motion which was set forth in the premises. It would seem, in short, that the key to the pathology is supplied by the physiology, and that the physiology is confirmed and established by the pathology. It is the same story throughout.

The treatment of spasm.

If the previous conclusion respecting the pathology of spasmodic disorders be correct, it is evident that antiphlogistic measures will hold no very prominent place in a sound plan of treatment. It is even probable that such measures will be as little wanted as they were in the treatment of convulsion or tremor. And certainly there is no evidence to the contrary in the results of past experience.

In catalepsy, a hot bath, enemas of hot wine and water, ether, and other remedies which will rouse the system, with tonics and restoratives in the intervals, will be the measures in which most persons would put their trust. Of this there can be little doubt.

"In all cases," says Dr. Watson, in his remarks upon the treatment of tetanus, "I should be more inclined to administer wine in large doses, and nutriment, than any particular drug," and this, I take it, is also the opinion of not a few of the soundest practitioners of this country. Many cases also are now on record in which the beneficial results of chloroform inhalations have been rendered evident, in relieving the pains as well as the spasms, and if care be taken to pour in wine and nourishment at the same time, there would seem to be no better plan. Another remedy, which will in all probability be found to be of great use, perhaps indispensable, is quinine. In some cases, it may be well to divide the nerve proceeding from the wound; but this measure is not likely to be required very often, particularly if the wine and food and quinine have been given vigorously, and the chloroform used judiciously, from the very beginning.

A similar line of treatment would also seem to be required in cholera, though here it is not likely that much good will be done by it unless the disease is taken in time. It is necessary, unhappily, not to be too sanguine as to the powers of medicine in the fully formed collapse; but there is no reason to doubt as to the practicability of preventing the disease by timely measures, even where the locality is highly unfavourable. At any rate, it is possible to prevent a disease which is in many respects analogous to cholera and not less deadly—the remittent fever of the West Coast of Africa—by giving, night and morning, a good dose of quinine in wine. With quinine and wine, indeed, it is possible to live for weeks and months, where without the quinine and wine a residence of a few hours might lead to a fatal result.

Nor is there any reason to suppose that a different line of treatment is required for the relief of the symptoms of ergotism.

The rigidity of cerebral paralysis, in all probability, is an irremediable evil. If the cerebral mischief is irreparable, and the power of using the muscles voluntarily is lost irrecoverably, the paralysed muscles, sooner or later, will pass into the state of "late rigidity;" and all that may be done is to defer the advent of this state by exercising the muscles with a galvanic current. Or if there is anything unusually inconvenient in the manner of the contraction, it may be necessary to consider the question of an operation by the subcutaneous method. Where the case is one of " early rigidity," the best treatment is perhaps that which does as little as possible. At any rate, after what has been said already, it can scarcely be necessary to have recourse to any kind of depletion.

In inflammation of the spinal cord or its membranes, chronic or acute, or in spinal apoplexy, the treatment must be guided by the same principles as those which were laid down when speaking of the corresponding affections of the brain.

In the treatment of the minor forms of spasmodic disorder, a main point will be to remove any local cause of irritation, such as carious teeth, worms, and so on. In other cases, of a more chronic character, the aid of the surgeon may not be unfrequently wanted in order to divide the contracted muscles. And if any general treatment is required, it may be supposed that they will be successful in proportion as it departs from anything of an antiphlogistic character. I know, for example, of four cases where attacks of laryngismus stridulus, which had frequently recurred under a treatment in which it had been thought essential to " regulate the secretions" by grey powder and so on, were put a stop to once and for all by a tonic and restorative plan of treatment— wine, beef-tea, steel, chloric ether; and I can speak with confidence of the beneficial results of a similar plan of treatment in a considerable number of cases of hooping-cough.

CPSIA information can be obtained
at www.ICGtesting.com
Printed in the USA
LVOW10*2304070518
576389LV00008B/58/P